SCHOOL OF ADVANCED STUDY UNIVERSITY OF LONDON
Institute of Germanic & Romance Studies

Constance Pascal (1877–1937)
Authority, Femininity and Feminism in French Psychiatry

igrs books

Established by the Institute of Germanic & Romance Studies, this series aims to bring to the public monographs and collections of essays in the field of modern foreign languages. Proposals for publication are selected by the Institute's editorial board, which is advised by a peer review committee of 36 senior academics in the field. To make titles as accessible as possible to an English-speaking and multi-lingual readership, volumes are written in English and quotations given in English translation.

For further details on the annual competition, visit:
http://www.igrs.sas.ac.uk/publications/igrs-books/igrs-books-annual-competition

igrs books Volume 8

Volume Editor

Professor Naomi Segal

Constance Pascal (1877–1937)
Authority, Femininity and Feminism in French Psychiatry

by

Felicia Gordon

SCHOOL OF ADVANCED STUDY UNIVERSITY OF LONDON

Institute of Germanic & Romance Studies

2013

Published by the

Institute of Germanic & Romance Studies
School of Advanced Study, University of London
Senate House, Malet Street, London WC1E 7HU
http://igrs.sas.ac.uk

Cover image
Constance Pascal *c.* 1925

First published 2013

ISBN 978 0 85457 236 6

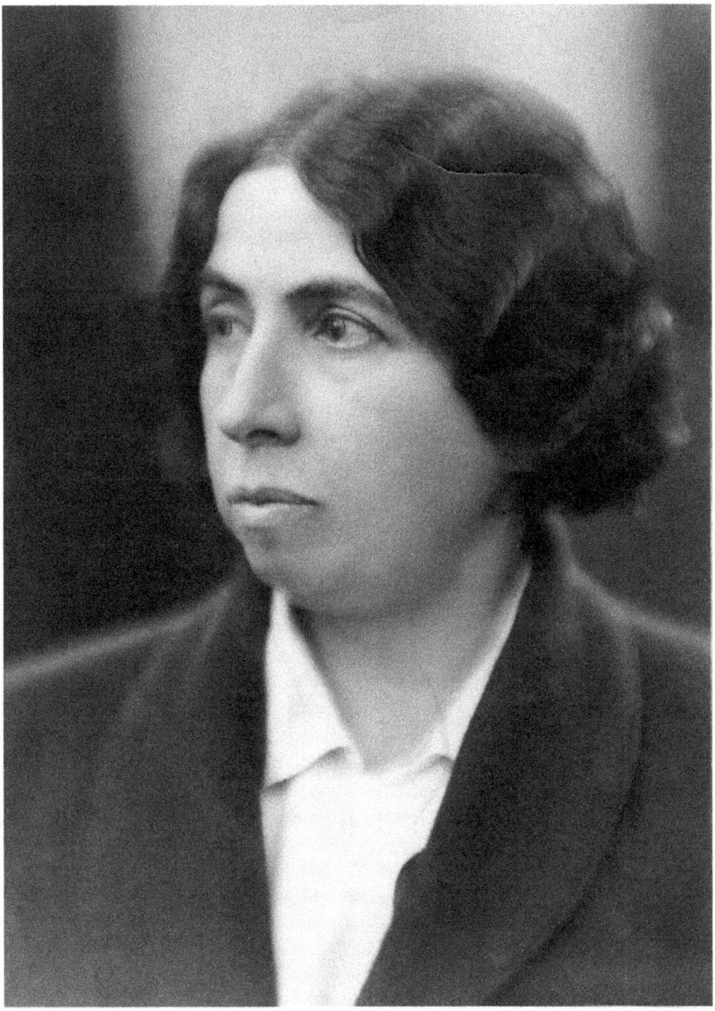

Constance Pascal c. *1925*

Contents

This book is dedicated to the memory of
Jeanne Pascal Rees.

Acknowledgements

I wish to thank the following libraries and archives for their assistance: Archives Historiques de la Ministère de Défense, Armée de la Terre, Vincennes; Archives de la Marne; Archives Nationales Fontainebleau, Centre des Archives Contemporaines; Archives de la Ville de Paris; Bibliothèque Charcot; Bibliothèque Historique de la Ville de Paris; Bibliothèque Marguerite Durand; Bibliothèque Nationale; Cambridge University Library; Centre Hospitalier de Clermont de l'Oise; Centre Hospitalier de Maison Blanche; Centre Hospitalier de Moisselles; Centre Hospitalier de Prémontré; Fonds Marie Louise Bouglé; Pascal/Rees Family Papers; the Wellcome Library.

I am most grateful to the Anglia Ruskin University, the British Academy and the Wellcome Trust for grants in support of this project.

I wish to thank the following for permission to use or reproduce material from articles previously published on Constance Pascal: Sage Publications Ltd, for an article in *History of Psychiatry*, 17 (2), June 2006; Taylor and Francis Group for an article on Madeleine Pelletier and Constance Pascal in *Modern and Contemporary France*, 17 (3) August 2009, see www.informaworld.com.

This book partly owes its existence to the family archive amassed by Jeanne Pascal Rees. I wish to thank warmly her daughter, Margaret Rees, who has been a continuing source of support and information. I am immensely grateful to the many friends and colleagues who have been generous with their time and constructive advice: Christine Bard, German Berrios, Clarissa Campbell Orr, Máire Cross, Monique and Paul Degèz, Jenny Fellowes, Véronique Fournier, Martin Garrett, Neil Hunt, Robert Inglesfield, Véronique Leroux-Hugon, Solange Mons, Karen Offen, Jane Rendall, Alison Sinclair and Conrad Smith. I wish particularly to thank Michel Caire for making Pascal's Maison Blanche papers available to me and for his illuminating discussion of her career. Richard J. Evans, who first persuaded me to embark on archival research in France, has consistently encouraged my work and been a wonderful example of scholarship to try to emulate. I owe a great debt both to Christine Corton and to my husband, Ian Gordon, who have read and commented on earlier drafts and offered sane and cheering counsel. I wish to thank Mary Orr of Southampton University for her advice on the text and Naomi Segal of Birkbeck, University of London, for her editorial guidance and her invaluable help in translating French texts. I am grateful to Jane Lewin at the Institute of Germanic & Romance Studies and the production team at the School of Advanced Study for their preparation of the printed text.

List of Illustrations

All images are reproduced by kind permission of Margaret Rees.

Abbreviations and Textual Notes

Throughout this book all translations, unless otherwise attributed, are my own and reference is given to the original text. Further references to a cited text will appear after quotations; passages without page reference are from the last-cited page, and page numbers without specified text are similarly from the last one named. Unless otherwise stated, all italics are the author's. Abbreviated titles used for archival sources and texts cited in this book are given below in alphabetical order of abbreviation. Full details can be found in the Bibliography.

AHMD	Archives Historiques de la Ministère de Défense, Armée de la Terre, Vincennes
AM	Archives de la Marne
AVP	Archives de la Ville de Paris
BMD	Bibliothèque Marguerite Durand
CAC	Archives Nationales, Centre des Archives Contemporaines de Fontainebleau
Clermont DACP	Centre Hospitalier de Clermont de l'Oise: Dossier Administratif Constance Pascal
CP	Constance Pascal
DJM	Dossier Justin Mengin
FMLB	Fonds Marie Louise Bouglé, Bibliothèque Historique de la Ville de Paris
IJPR	Interviews with Jeanne Pascal Rees
MBDACP	Centre Hospitalier de Maison Blanche: Dossier Administratif Constance Pascal
Moisselles DACP	Centre Hospitalier de Moisselles: Dossier Administratif Constance Pascal
Prémontré DACP	Centre Hospitalier de Prémontré: Dossier Administratif Constance Pascal
PRFP	Pascal/Rees Family Papers

1. Introduction

This biography traces the life and career of Constance Pascal (1877–1937), the first woman in France to become a fully qualified psychiatrist. I first became aware of Pascal in 1989 when writing a book on the medical, feminist and political career of Madeleine Pelletier who, in 1903, campaigned for women to be allowed to sit the examination for psychiatric interns from which they had formerly been excluded. Both she and Pascal sat and passed, giving them initial entry into the state funded psychiatric profession. I had noted Pascal's name, but had remarked that, unlike Pelletier, she 'made no pretensions to feminist sympathies'.[1] These attributes, I inferred, had, in the generally conservative gender culture of France, made possible her successful career. As I came to realize, this was a very partial assessment. While it is true that Pascal was praised for her feminine and maternal presence, she also displayed a combative attitude to higher authority and a deep commitment to women's advancement throughout her career.

Pascal was again drawn to my attention on 7 November 2001 when I received a courteous letter from a Mme Jeanne Pascal Rees, living in Oxford, enclosing an article she had written on Pascal who, it transpired, was her mother.[2] Through the ensuing correspondence, interviews and friendship that grew up between us, I discovered the

1 Felicia Gordon, *The Integral Feminist: Madeleine Pelletier, 1874–1939* (Cambridge: Polity Press, 1990), 70–71. Charles Sowerwine, 'Madeleine Pelletier, femme, médecin, militante', *L'Information psychiatrique*, 9 (1988), 1189 and Felicia Gordon, though mentioning Pascal's career, focused primarily on journalistic eulogies to her beauty and femininity, largely overlooking her psychiatric and feminist achievements. We have since both revised our views. See Felicia Gordon, 'French Psychiatry and the new woman: the case of Dr Constance Pascal', *History of Psychiatry*, 17 (2) (2006), 159–82.

2 Jeanne Rees, 'À propos de Constance Pascal, première femme aliéniste en France', *L'Information psychiatrique*, 2 (2001), 173–84, hereafter abbreviated 'ÀPCP'.

remarkable story of Pascal, who had pursued a highly successful psychiatric career, while maintaining secrecy over her illegitimate daughter. The contradictions that Pascal experienced between her brilliant career and her maternal devotion were, as Jeanne Rees argued, a sad and moving reflection on the social history of the period. Although one of the dangers of personal testimony is the fashioning of a hagiographic account, Jeanne Rees's case exemplifies her remarkable capacity for objectivity. This, coupled with evidence from Pascal's letters, journal and official dossiers, reveals her combative personality and sometimes difficult personal relations and ensures a more nuanced view.

In her determination to preserve her mother's memory, Mme Rees amassed an extensive family archive, referred to here as the Pascal Rees Family Papers (PRFP). Although Pascal's professional career had been extensively examined by Jean-Michel Barbier, prior to Mme Rees granting me access to her family archive, virtually no information on her personal life had been available.[3] Though sources in any biography, no matter how well known the individual, are always necessarily partial and incomplete, in many ways the gaps in the record can be as significant as the episodes fully documented. The sources that underpin this biography are both personal and official. Personal sources include: the recollections that Jeanne Rees made available to me, both oral and written; Pascal's journal and letters to family members in her native Romania; a variety of official documents; press interviews; an unpublished play/film script; and family photographs. Constance Pascal's letters to her brother, Trajan Pascal, offer glimpses of her youthful rebellion against her assumed destiny as a marriageable girl of good family. The film script, '*La Goutte de sang*' [The Drop of Blood], is one of the most personally revealing documents of this multi-talented woman. In the official category are the administrative dossiers at the five psychiatric hospitals where she worked; the summative administrative dossier in the Centre des Archives Contemporaines at Fontainebleau, including correspondence with ministers; her extensive psychiatric publications; and archival material relating to her naturalization and to the career of General Justin Mengin, the father of her child. Among the gaps, such as the lack of documentation on Pascal's childhood, the most telling must be her destruction of some of her journal entries and of her correspondence with her family in Romania, and what

3 Jean-Michel Barbier, 'La vie et l'œuvre de Constance Pascal (1877–1937)', Thèse pour le Doctorat en Médecine, Diplôme d'Etat (Université de Picardie: Faculté de Médicine d'Amiens, 9 January 1997).

this reveals about her emotional conflicts. Nonetheless, this web of personal and objective sources has made it possible both to construct the portrait of a complex and brilliant individual, who experienced the possibilities open to, and limitations operating on, women in France at the beginning of the twentieth century, and to evaluate her contribution to psychiatry and feminism.

Constance Pascal was one of a number of women intellectuals who migrated to western Europe in the late nineteenth and early twentieth centuries, often described as 'new women', in search of higher education and entry into the professions.[4] These young pioneers represented part of a larger trend concerning women's aspirations, but they were also exceptional and atypical members of their generation, through their ambition, intellectual gifts and relatively privileged class position. Pascal's literal journey from Romania to France, her geographical and cultural displacement, may indeed have given her particular empathy with the mentally disoriented patients in the psychiatric hospitals where she worked for over thirty years. The story of her life, experiencing and challenging the constraints of custom and convention, reveals the characteristic patterns, opportunities and limitations of life for women in France from the *fin de siècle* to the beginnings of the Second World War.

Both in her life and in her profession, Constance straddled several seemingly antithetical worlds: eastern and western Europe; the life of the leisured landed gentry and the work-oriented life of the professional classes; genteel lady and professional woman; respectable *bourgeoise* and single mother. We see her attempting, as a psychiatrist, to bridge the chasm between the mental worlds of her patients and psychiatry's rationalising structures. One finds in her private and professional writing a consciousness of the fragility of rationality. A key aspect of her life story is the way it illustrates conflicts arising for women between professional ambition and private life. The fact that nothing has emerged about her personal history until recently indicates Constance's overriding need to appear in her profession as a psychiatrist first and last, to conceal the personal from the public gaze – not only out of a love of privacy, but because for a woman in a hitherto all-male profession, any laxity or

4 See Linda L. Clark, *Women and Achievement in Nineteenth-Century Europe* (Cambridge: Cambridge University Press, 2008), 1–8; Mary Louise Roberts, *Civilization without Sexes: Reconstructing Gender in Post-War France, 1917–1927* (Chicago and London: University of Chicago Press, 1994); Mary Louise Roberts, *Disruptive Acts: The New Woman in* Fin-de-Siècle *France* (Chicago and London: University of Chicago Press, 2002).

irregularity in her personal life would have left her open to censure and disgrace in a way unimaginable for male colleagues.

Hers can therefore be construed as a story of elites, of a woman of unusual abilities who succeeded in a competitive field. Yet she devoted her life to some of society's most marginalized and inarticulate people, the insane of the hospitals where she worked. She championed the nurses in the asylums in which she was stationed, and argued for improvements in training, pay and conditions. She battled to set up schools for mentally and physically handicapped children, who were 'warehoused' in psychiatric hospitals. Her commitment to her patients shines through private letters and official reports.

Traditional biography or life-writing, because of its assumptions of a progressive narrative, was legitimately questioned in the critical climate of the late 1950s. Major challenges to scholarly biographical writing arose at this time with a return to a purely empirical, non-theoretical approach to describing political or social change. A positivist orientation continued in the decentring of individual experience by economic and social historians, pioneered by Fernand Braudel, editor of the journal *Annales* from 1956 to 1968.[5] This unpeopled and almost static history showed the determining effects of structures on individuals whose consciousnesses were tied to superficial events and thus painted an illusory picture of the world. Narratives of individual achievement, such as traditional biography, were, in this interpretation, largely irrelevant. Equally undermining for traditional ideas of biographical writing was the challenge thrown out by the poststructuralist critique of subjective coherence, including Derrida's rejection of the hermeneutic project. If there is no stable centre of self, and if interpretation of actions is random and subjective, biography, since at the simplest level it seeks to construct life as a narrative, becomes an impossible project. Though this is not a new perception – memorably tackled in fiction by Laurence Sterne in *The Life and Opinions of Tristram Shandy, Gentleman* in the eighteenth century and by Sartre in *La Nausée* in the twentieth – it is reasonable to ask whether writing the narrative of a life as a coherent or interpretable whole can be validated as part of any larger historical project.[6] The mere fact that stories are popular does not

5 Stuart Clark, 'The *Annales historians*', in *The Return of Grand Theory in the Human Sciences*, Quentin Skinner (ed.) (Cambridge: Cambridge University Press), 179–96.

6 See Consuelo Corradi, 'Text, context and individual meaning: rethinking life stories in a hermeneutic framework', *Discourse and Society*, 2: 1 (1991), 105–18; Marlene Kadar, *Essays on Life Writing* (Toronto and London: University of Toronto Press, 1992); Alanson Lloyd Moote, 'New bottles and new wine: The

make them historically valuable.[7] Yet every individual conceives of his or her life on some level as a narrative; that is how life is lived. However fictitious or illusory, the desire for narrative coherence worked out over time appears central to human experience.[8] As Jo Burr Margadant has suggested, it is more helpful to think of biography in terms of the politics of identity construction. Here the biographical subject is a multiple self, performed over time to create a fictive or willed coherence out of conflicting selves or roles.[9] It is this heterogeneity, connected by memory, that Proust celebrates in *Le Temps retrouvé* [*Time Regained*]:

> [...] ne manquerais-je pas d'abord d'y décrire les hommes (cela dût-il les faire ressembler à des êtres monstrueux) comme occupant une place si considérable, à côté de celle si restreinte qui leur est réservée dans l'espace, une place au contraire prolongée sans mesure – puisqu'ils touchent simultanément, comme des géants plongés dans les années, à des époques si distantes, entre lesquelles tant de jours sont venus se placer – dans le Temps.[10]

> [[...] I should not fail, even if the results were to make them resemble monsters, to describe men first and foremost as occupying a place, a very considerable place compared with the restricted one which is allotted to them in space, a place on the contrary prolonged past measure – for simultaneously, like giants plunged into the years, they

current state of early modernist biographical writing', *French Historical Studies*, 19: 4 (1996), 911–26. For an assessment of postmodernist theory in relation to the writing of history see Richard J. Evans, *In Defence of History* (London: Granta Books, 1997).

7 'As opposed to all forms of fiction, biography and autobiography are referential texts: exactly like scientific or historical discourse, they claim to provide information about a "reality" exterior to the text, and so to submit to a test of verification', Philippe Lejeune, *On Autobiography* [*Le Pacte autobiographique*, 1975], trans. Katherine Leary (Minneapolis: University of Minnesota Press, 1989), 22. For further exploration of narrative-truth problems associated with autobiography and biography see Philippe Lejeune (ed.), *Le Désir biographique* (Paris: Université de Paris X, 1988).

8 The issue of subjectivity to validate the objective world is relevant in Bergson's 'solution' for Xeno's paradox of motion: Henri Bergson, *Essai sur les données immédiates de la conscience* (Paris: Alcan, 1901).

9 Jo Burr Margadant (ed.), *The New Biography: Performing Femininity in Nineteenth-Century France* (Berkeley and London: University of California Press, 2000), 7.

10 Marcel Proust (1927), *À la recherche du temps perdu* (Paris: Gallimard, 1954), 1167.

touch epochs that are immensely far apart, separated by the slow accretion of many, many days – in the dimension of Time.][11]

Nevertheless, as long as it remains within historical disciplines, biography should not merely record self-constructions and multiple identities, but their relevance to and conflicts with the social world in which the individual subject lived. History should not be confused with memory, but requires the critical interrogation of memory, and of the myths the latter generates.[12] In the case of Constance Pascal, her profession as a psychiatrist in French state asylums brought her into daily contact with patients who had seemingly lost all inner coherence or who, in order to retain their sense of themselves, rejected the view of the world called reality held by the majority of people, a sort of über-Derridean, post-interpretative state, namely madness. Pascal, whose career was devoted to empirical science and whose early training was in the positivist climate of French scientism, never abandoned her commitment to objective scientific enquiry. However, in the course of a professional life stretching from 1906 to 1937, her interest shifted from largely nosological analyses of mental illness (categorization according to external symptoms), typical of the profession in the late nineteenth and early twentieth centuries, to a search for therapeutic interventions via shock therapy, and ultimately to a focus on the patients' subjective suffering, rather than on the external manifestations or symptoms displayed in their illness. Like Julia Kristeva (also an Eastern European immigrant to France) a generation later, Pascal recognized that the 'sorrows of love' could be a precipitating trauma for a loss of self, producing in Kristeva's words, 'un vertige d'identité' [a giddiness of identity].[13]

In validating the reality of subjective suffering in her patients – predominantly women – Pascal's work, while still rigorously empirical, demonstrates the influence of Bergson, Proust and Freud, particularly in her last monograph, *Chagrins d'amour et psychoses* [The Sorrows of Love and Psychosis].[14] Her recourse to a modified form

11 Marcel Proust, *Remembrance of Things Past,* vol. III (1927), trans. C. K. Scott Moncrieff, T. Kilmartin and A. Mayor (Harmondsworth: Penguin, 1981), 1107.

12 Richard J. Evans, 'The Tory Interpretation of History', *London Review of Books*, 33: 6 (17 March 2011), 12.

13 Constance Pascal, *Chagrins d'amour et psychoses* [1935] (Paris: L'Harmattan, 2000). Julia Kristeva, *Histoires d'amour* (Paris: Denoël, 1983), 11.

14 On psychology and subjectivity see Annick Ohayon, *L'Impossible Rencontre: psychologie et psychanalyse en France 1919–1969* (Paris: Editions de la Découverte, 1999); Thomas Hardy Leahey, *A History of Psychology: Main Currents in Psychological Thought* (Upper Saddle River, NJ: Prentice Hal, 2000); Théodore

of psychoanalysis led her – like the founder of psychoanalysis – to endeavour to discover the narrative of a patient's life (for those who often had lost the power of speech or coherence) buried under the seemingly inexplicable symptoms of 'mad' behaviour. Signalling what for her was the salient aspect of his work, Pascal wrote:

> Un autre grand mérite de Freud est de nous avoir appris à regarder derrière les aspects cliniques et à découvrir la souffrance jusqu'à la racine des instincts. Il nous a expliqué pourquoi il fallait se méfier du 'signe', ombre pâle, reflet changeant de la libido traquée qui se dérobe (*CAP*, 56).

> [Another of Freud's great merits is to have taught us to look behind clinical symptoms and discover the suffering at the very root of the instincts. He has explained why one must distrust the 'sign', that pale shadow, that shifting reflection of the hounded libido which is so difficult to see.]

A journalist who followed her work called her 'le plus doux des détectives' [the gentlest of detectives].[15] Yet Pascal knew that unmediated recollections, while they served in Proust's 'admirable étude psychologique et littéraire' [admirable psychological and literary study] (*CAP*, 99) to reintegrate the narrator's multiple selves, could also become, in the less fortunate, a source of psychosis. 'Le blessé d'amour souffre parce qu'il se souvient' [A person wounded by love suffers because he remembers] (*CAP*, 159).

A study of Pascal's career is therefore also a biography of her times and entails a consideration of the development of French psychiatry from the *Belle Époque* to the eve of the Second World War. Her prolific publications constitute a record not only of her own research but of the evolution of French psychiatric theory and practice. Although much of the technical terminology in those writings is now obsolete, or has been superseded, the tragic human conditions represented in them remain. Alongside this technical vocabulary, one sometimes finds, shockingly, the casual terms employed by professionals and the public alike to refer to people with enduring mental health conditions. 'Abnormals' [*anormaux*], 'degenerates', 'imbeciles', 'cretins', 'lunatics', 'the mad' [*aliénés*] were commonly used terms. They demonstrate how a multiplicity of neurological impairments

Ribot, *Les Maladies de la mémoire* (Paris: Germer Beullière, 1881); *Les Maladies de la personnalité* (Paris: Germer Beullière, 1885); *Problèmes de psychologie affective* (Paris: Alcan, 1910); Frédéric Paulhan, *La Fonction de la mémoire et le souvenir affectif* (Paris: Félix Alcan, 1904).

15 Louis Roubaud, 'Démons et déments', *Détective* (December, 1932), 5.

were lumped together in the psychiatric hospitals of the day, just as epileptics were routinely incarcerated in asylums with the severely mentally ill. These phenomena also reflect the popular fear and contempt that psychiatric disorders have always aroused. To her immense credit, Pascal sought to demystify her patients' illnesses to the public through interviews in the mainstream press. She opened a window on the treatment and sufferings of the mentally ill in the first half of the twentieth century.

This biography makes no claim to psychoanalyse its subject. It draws attention, however, to Pascal's recognition that maintaining a coherent self in the face of both internal and external discords, while possible for the strong-willed like herself, proved too great a challenge for the many patients populating France's huge asylums. Whereas in regard to her *aliénés* (the French word foregrounds the idea of separation from the self), she strove to restore them to themselves, to detoxify their memories; she seems, when dealing with her own mental and emotional conflicts, to have attempted to cauterize memory. She cut herself off from her Romanian family for long periods, partly in an effort to forget her past, and chose to foreclose the memorialization of her own life by her psychiatric colleagues. To understand or interpret this 'forgetting' is one of the aims of this study. As Quentin Skinner observes: 'The explanation of human action must include an attempt to recover and interpret the meanings of social actions from the point of view of the agents performing them' (*Return*, 6). To the extent that Pascal engaged in a hermeneutic study of her patients, it seems appropriate to attempt a similar task with regard to her self-fashioning, her self-performance as a feminine, but authoritative, professional woman. Though highly individual, it was also derived from available cultural models.

Constance Pascal was representative of that pre-First World War, pan-European society of the well-educated and generally well-born, not unlike the society chronicled by Proust, whom she so admired. Her Romanian family of impoverished gentry formed part of a predominately Francophile culture. Although living in a still feudal society, Pascal absorbed, paradoxically, the ethos of the Enlightenment, veneration for France and for the values of the Third Republic. Her rebellion against her stultifying family background, her hunger for education, her attachment to the politics of French anti-clericalism and of the Left link her to the many ambitious women who left Eastern Europe for the freer intellectual climate of

Switzerland and France.[16] On one level, this biography, which traces Pascal's ambition to enter the medical and psychiatric professions, links her to early French feminism in the context of women's entry into the professions. On another level it follows the permutations of French psychiatric theory and practice in the course of her career and asks to what extent she challenged or was compliant with the dominant ethos informing asylum-care. Pascal's personal history is crucial to any understanding of her complex personality, her alienation from her Romanian family and her determination to nurture and educate her illegitimate daughter. The extent to which these tensions impacted on her psychiatric theory and practice and on the persona she projected to the world help to explain the narrative she constructed of her multi-stranded life.

As a biographical subject, Pascal presents the reader with fruitful dichotomies: assurance and anguish, high public profile and deeply protected privacy. Given her background in the Romanian landed gentry, she possessed considerable class assurance, while hating the stagnant life of enforced lady-like leisure mapped out for her by her family. After she had emigrated from Romania to France, though steeped in francophone culture from an early age, she nevertheless had to fight for acceptance, both as a foreigner and, particularly in her profession, as a woman. On the one hand her public, professional image was authoritative and assured: on the other, she was often anguished, overwhelmed by work and responsibilities and, though she rejoiced in the birth of her daughter, possessive and obsessed with the need she felt to make up for the child's illegitimate status by a rigorous academic education. While she maintained a complete separation between her public and private roles, Pascal did not shun the limelight. From the outset of her medical-psychiatric career she gave press interviews and featured, because of her charm, poise and appealing looks, as the acceptable face of modernity for women in the professions.[17]

Pascal's determination to be forgotten after her death constitutes a particularly interesting biographical conundrum, compounded by her own veto over memorialization. Her erasure until recently from psychiatric and women's history arose from a number of factors:

16 See Thomas Neville Bonner, *To the Ends of the Earth: Women's Search for Education in Medicine* (Cambridge, MA: Harvard University Press, 1991), 49–75; Linda Clark, *Women and Achievement*, 171–217; Mary R. S. Creese, *Ladies in the Laboratory II* (Lanham, MD: The Scarecrow Press, 2004), 57–97.

17 Felicia Gordon, 'Publicity and Professionalism: Madeleine Pelletier (1874–1939) and Constance Pascal (1877–1937)', *Modern and Contemporary France*, 17: 3 (2009), 319–34.

the technical difficulty of her psychiatric writing; changes in the terminology of the psychiatric illnesses in which she had specialized; the post-war reaction in France to inter-war psychiatry following the Vichy era; and the erroneous impression among historians that she was not a feminist.[18] Her daughter, Mme Jeanne Pascal Rees, was resolved to see her mother's achievements publicly remembered before her own death in 2006. Jeanne Pascal Rees's breadth of vision, intelligence and compassion for both her parents as actors in a complex web of historical circumstance, are a tribute to her and to her mother's unstinting devotion.

In Constance Pascal we witness the interplay of individual agency and historical circumstance played out in a fiercely ambitious, brilliant and emotionally driven woman. She can appear most compelling if not always sympathetic, when confronting the crises of her life. Her particular story illuminates French psychiatric theory and practice of the period, throws fresh light on the social mores of domestic ideology in the Third Republic and on key aspects of French feminism. It is a moving story of courage, compassion and the steely determination characteristic of a generation of women intellectuals breaking into and conquering the professions. Women's history, which has rescued many women from historical obscurity, has no need to apologize for commemorating the lives of individuals as they lived, were shaped by and reacted to their historical moment. We see in Constance Pascal someone who constructed her chosen roles, sometimes imperfectly and against the grain, but with extraordinary dedication and an ironic perception of herself as performing on a tightrope of gendered expectations.

18 Pascal's career was first examined by Jean Michel Barbier in his doctoral thesis of 1997 and subsequently by Barbier, Gérard Serra and Gwenolé Loas, 'Constance Pascal: pioneer of French psychiatry', *History of Psychiatry*, 10 (1999), 425–37. Barbier was unable to discover anything about her private life. Mme Jeanne Pascal Rees, 'ÀPCP', 173–83, first revealed the story of her parents' relationship and gave valuable background on Pascal's Romanian origins. For psychiatry and the Vichy period, see Isabelle von Buelzingsloewen, *L'Hécatombe des fous: la famine dans les hôpitaux psychiatriques français sous l'Occupation* (Paris: Aubier, 2007) and N. Henckes, 'Réformer et soigner: l'émergence de la psychothérapie institutionnelle en France, 1944–1955', *Psychiatries dans l'histoire* (Caen: PUC, 2008), 277–88.

2. Between Two Worlds, 1877–1908

On an icy morning in late December 1937 in the cemetery of Neuilly sur Marne on the eastern outskirts of Paris, a small group of mourners gathered to watch a coffin being lowered into its grave. Following the deceased's instructions, there was no religious ceremony. Dr Constance Pascal, consultant psychiatrist at the Maison Blanche Asylum, was attended at her burial by her daughter Jeanne, her oldest friend Mlle Jeanne Streicher and a handful of staff from the hospital. Returning to the villa on the edge of the hospital grounds, where she had lived with her mother and had seen her die, twenty-one-year-old Jeanne Pascal arranged for the two family dogs to be destroyed, as her mother had requested. Then, having no further right of domicile in the tied house at the hospital, she went to lodge with Mlle Streicher, who saw it as her mission to ensure that her namesake, Jeanne Pascal, pass her examinations for the *agrégation,* leading to a qualification as *lycée* teacher.[1]

Constance Pascal's iron will and formidable intelligence, passed on to her daughter, would serve the latter well. However, the story behind Constance Pascal's bleak funeral, her adamant refusal to allow eulogistic obituaries in the psychiatric press and her near-disappearance from the historical record encapsulates both the extraordinary professional dedication of the first woman in France to become a fully qualified psychiatrist and the secrecy she preserved about her private life.[2] The absolute division Pascal maintained between her private and public worlds, though particular to her situation as a professional woman and an unmarried mother, was also symptomatic of constraints on women entering hitherto all-

1 Jeanne Pascal Rees, 'Maladie et mort de Constance Pascal, juin–décembre 1937', MS, PRFP (2003).

2 The one short obituary, appearing in print, was by Pascal's colleague, Jacques Vié, 'Nécrologie Mlle C. Pascal (1877–1937)', *Annales medico-psychologiques,* 2 (1937), 788 and 868; reprinted in *La Presse médicale* (January 1938), 150.

male professions. Pascal's life story offers a glimpse of the conflicts undergone and the opportunities seized by talented women in France during and after the *Belle Époque*.

When in 1897 Constanza Pascal,[3] a native of Romania, obtained permission from her family to pursue her medical studies abroad, France was the country to which she naturally turned. The opening up of medical training in France to women in 1868 had not produced a flood of French applicants, however. In an initial cohort of four women, only one, Mme Brès, was French.[4] Young French women of the bourgeoisie, in general, remained attached to the ideological expectations of their class that they would become wives and mothers.[5] Yet in spite of gender expectations for bourgeois women still firmly rooted in domestic ideology, in the labour market women had begun to enter the professions, not in large, but still in significant numbers.[6] France, which had opened its universities and medical schools to women at a time when in Britain, the United States and much of Europe they were still excluded, was a beacon of opportunity to talented women.

Constance Pascal formed part of a significant foreign intake into French higher education that continued even after the turn of the century. Many of these young women gravitated to medicine. For them, cultural norms and male anxieties about gender must have seemed mild in relation to the still rigid class- and gender-structures of their own countries. Though within France the image of the 'new woman', abandoning domestic life for a career in traditionally male fields, was deemed threatening to sections of the male bourgeoisie, the actual numbers were extremely small. In *France and Women* James

3 She was christened 'Constanza' but had Gallicized her name to 'Constance' by the turn of the century.

4 The other three were English (Miss Garrett), American (Miss Putnam) and Russian (Mlle Gontcharoff). The foreign intake continued to be high even after the turn of the century (Gordon, *IF*), 28.

5 See Edmée Charrier, *L'Évolution intellectuelle féminine* (Paris: Librairie du Recueil Sirey, 1937); Françoise Mayeur, *L'Éducation des filles en France au XIXe siècle* (Paris: Hachette, 1979) and James F. McMillan, *Housewife or Harlot, The Place of Women in French Society, 1870–1940* (Brighton: Harvester, 1981).

6 For the importance of domestic ideology in nineteenth-century France see Susan K. Grogan, *French Socialism and Sexual Difference: Women and the New Society 1803–44* (Basingstoke: Macmillan, 1992); Mary Louise Roberts, *Civilization without Sexes;* James F. McMillan, *France and Women 1789–1914: Gender, Society and Politics* (London and New York: Routledge, 2000). For a sociological and feminist reading of the professions see Anne Witz, *Professions and Patriarchy* (London: Routledge, 1992).

F. McMillan points to the slow progress of women's access to higher education and the professions once these were open to them.[7] In the years before 1914, female representation in the professions was 0.29% for law, 3% for doctors, 8% for dentists, 3% for pharmacists and 2.6% for chemists and engineers. The proportion of French women students exceeded that of foreigners for the first time only in 1912–13. While, on the one hand, this may demonstrate the grip of domestic ideology, it also shows that France was a beacon of opportunity for foreign women. Fortunately for them, perhaps, foreigners could be viewed through French eyes as exceptions to the rule of obligatory femininity and domesticity. Still, whether French-born or foreign, women entering higher education and the professions assumed a symbolic importance out of all proportion to their statistical mass. These women saw themselves – and were seen – as role models, pioneers and rebels.

As a medical student at the turn of the century, Constance Pascal can be construed as a 'new woman' by virtue of her remarkable spirit of independence and her desire to succeed, though it is doubtful whether she would have accepted the epithet for herself. Whereas the 'new woman' was often seen as flouting convention in her love life, profession, dress sense or sporting ambitions (much was made of the liberating effects of the bicycle, especially in caricatures and cartoons), many ambitious women took care to avoid a flamboyant lifestyle, or indeed to rock the boat, in relation to gender roles.[8] Professions such as teaching, medicine and psychiatry demanded of women, even more than men, both dedication and social decorum. The advantages of secure conditions of service (a promotion ladder, statutory sick leave, annual holidays and pension rights) were often tempered by the sense of marginality and social isolation, as is well documented in the lives of *institutrices* [primary school teachers] and women *lycée* teachers.[9] Pascal, a woman striving to break into the newer professional élites, adopted a conventional feminine persona.[10] It is indicative of the importance of gender roles that the praise lavished on her by journalists in 1905 after her successful viva

7 McMillan, *France and Women*, 141–59.

8 For the subversive undermining of gender roles by the New Women, see Roberts, *Disruptive Acts*.

9 Jo Burr Margadant, *Madame le Professeur: Women Educators in the Third Republic* (Princeton: Princeton University Press, 1992), 4. Margadant argues that the first generation of women *lycée* teachers, an important professional group, was still closely tied to the French domestic ideal.

10 Roberts, *Civilisation*, 11.

for her doctoral thesis turned principally on her femininity, charm and grace.

Two of Pascal's closest friends when she was a student in Paris were *lycée* teachers. Mathilde Salomon (1837–1909) taught at the Collège Sévigné and Jeanne Streicher was one of the first women to become *agrégée* at the École Normale de Sévres.[11] Both were remarkable women. Françoise Mayeur notes that

> an extraordinary degree of tenacity and a genuinely exceptional talent were necessary if a woman were to succeed. If she lacked wealth or birth, a woman needed a network of friends and protectors: one thinks of Mathilde Salomon, who was the protégée of the republicans and was appointed director of the Collège Sévigné.[12]

Jeanne Streicher was also a product of the republic, a fervent believer in Cartesian ideals of reason and Kantian duty. She taught herself Latin and Greek in order to be able to tutor her pupils for the baccalaureate.[13] These women belonged to a generation whose professional lives were marked by devotion to public service and to the very republic that denied them full status as citizens. In her psychiatric calling, Pascal reflected the same values. If they were subversive in their simultaneous espousal of professional and domestic values, they avoided the flirtatious and occasionally scandalous behaviour of women like Marguerite Durand or Sarah Bernhardt.[14] In relation to her profession, Constance Pascal was what the French term 'très sérieuse' [deeply serious]. Such women enacted gender roles that were politically adventurous by breaking down barriers in the professions, but at the cost of always presenting an appearance of impeccable social and gender conformity. As Judith Butler suggests: 'The reproduction of the category of gender is enacted on a large political scale, as when women first enter a profession or

11 Streicher's dates are not known but she lived until at least 1958 when she published her study of the seventeenth-century poet Théophile de Viau.

12 Françoise Mayeur, 'Women and elites from the nineteenth to the twentieth century', ed. Loyon Howorth and Philip G. Cerny, *Elites in France: Origins, Reproduction and Power* (London: Frances Pinter, 1981), 60.

13 Jeanne Pascal Rees, 'Recollections of Jeanne Streicher', MS, PRFP.

14 Roberts, *Disruptive Acts*: 'They acted out various gender roles at a dizzying pace, merging them so fluidly as to contest their naturalised status. Thanks to their adventures, conventional femininity was exposed as a choice, not a destiny', 17.

gain certain rights, or are reconceived in legal or political discourse in significantly new ways'.[15]

If they were not overt rebels, these exceptional women nevertheless saw themselves as feminist innovators in the sense of opening their professions to other women and serving as role models for subsequent generations. Pascal's perception of this role emerges clearly in an article she wrote in 1933 on the competitive examination for asylum doctors, in which she notes, not without irony, the growing acceptability of women in psychiatry. Referring to the medieval scholastic debate as to women's full humanity, which tacitly underpinned the thinking of male professors at the time she qualified in 1908, Pascal rejoiced that more women were joining the profession:

> Ce concours a été surtout illustre par ses succès féministes. Trois femmes ont emporté la victoire, et j'espère la gloire. Trois femmes fonctionnaires de plus dans la société actuelle. C'est un record que le féminisme n'a pas encore battu au concours du médicat. À l'époque lointaine où je me suis présentée à l'adjuvant,[16] on discutait encore si la femme avait une âme. Au dernier concours, on ne discuta que la valeur des épreuves, et j'ai eu la conviction nette que si tous mes collègues n'étaient pas féministes, ils n'avaient aucune hostilité envers les candidates. La question professionnelle, utile aux femmes, qu'on a agitée, est la suivante: la femme peut-elle diriger un service

15 Judith Butler, 'Performative Acts and Gender Constitution: An Essay in Phenomenology and Feminist Theory', in *Performing Feminisms: Feminist Critical Theory and Theatre*, ed. Sue-Ellen Crane (Baltimore and London: Johns Hopkins University Press, 1990), 275. In *Gender Trouble: feminism and the subversion of identity* (New York and London: Routledge, 1999) Butler develops this argument much further, with aspects that could apply to Pascal; for example: 'Gender ought not to be constructed as a stable identity or locus of agency from which various acts follow; rather, gender is an identity tenuously constituted in time, instituted in an exterior space through the *stylized repetition of acts*'; and going further: 'If gender attributes and acts, the various ways in which a body shows or produces its cultural signification, are performative, then there is no pre-existing identity by which an act or attribute might be measured; there would be no true or false, real or distorted acts of gender, and the postulation of a true gender identity would be revealed as a regulatory fiction', 179–80.

16 Internships were posts for medical and psychiatry students still in training. The qualification for a psychiatric intern was success in the relevant 'concours' or competitive examination. On completion of the internship, as we saw with Pelletier and Pascal, interns applied for a permanent post in the psychiatric service, the lowest rung being the 'adjuvant' or 'poste de médecin adjoint'. The post of 'adjuvant' was the equivalent to that of junior doctor, though the candidate was fully trained. This lowest tier in the psychiatric hierarchy was eventually abolished.

> d'hommes? Or, j'ai débuté à Clermont dans un service d'hommes, ensuite j'ai dirigé à Prémontré un autre service d'hommes, à Châlons, à Moisselle où j'étais directrice, j'ai eu des hommes sous mes ordres. Jamais je n'ai eu à me plaindre de leur désobéissance.[17]

> [This competitive examination has above all been remarkable for its feminist success. Three women swept to victory and I hope fame. Three more women civil servants [*in this case, psychiatrists*] in present-day society. It is an unbeaten record by feminism in the *concours du médicat*. In the far-off period when I entered the [*competive examination for*] junior doctors, the question of whether or not women had souls was still under discussion. In this most recent exam, the only dispute was about the quality of the answers, and I had the strong conviction that, even if all my colleagues were not feminists, they were in no way hostile towards their female candidates. The professional question of concern to women candidates that was debated was the following: can a woman manage a male ward? I myself began my career at Clermont in a male ward, then I ran another male ward at Prémontré, and at Châlons and Moisselles, where I was the director, I had men working under my orders. I never had any problems with discipline.]

Pascal's enthusiasm at the advent of three more female colleagues was justifiable. Nevertheless, the number of women psychiatrists in 1933 had only risen to seven.[18] Still, this was an advance over the one woman in 1908 – Constance Pascal herself.

Here Pascal refutes the arguments of those like Dr Édouard Toulouse who, though a supporter of women's rights, had expressed fears that women psychiatrists would lack authority with male patients and staff. Indeed, though she may not have known it, she had once been accused of just such a failing.[19] Taking a contrary position from Toulouse, however, the socialist anthropologist Léonce Manouvrier had argued against the idea of the basic inferiority of women, a naked prejudice, he said, disguised as scientific objectivity. Pascal may have remembered his article of 1903:

> Des théologiens s'étaient demandés si la femme avait une âme. Des savants furent bien près, un certain nombre de siècles plus tard, de lui refuser une intelligence humaine. On peut lire dans les recueils

17 Constance Pascal, 'Réflexions sur le concours du médicat des asiles de 1933: Pourquoi le médecin aliéniste doit [*sic*] être polyvalent?' [Thoughts on the competitive examination for psychiatric hospital doctors, 1933: Why should psychiatrists be versatile?], MS, PRFP (1933).

18 I am indebted to Dr Michel Caire for this statistic from the *Annales médico-psychologiques* (January 1936).

19 Préfet de l'Oise, report on Constance Pascal, DCPCAC (9 March 1915).

scientifiques des plus estimées maintes réflexions et conclusions d'après lesquelles il semblait que, dans l'évolution de l'espèce humaine, la femme fût restée sous divers rapports des plus importants, notamment par son développement cérébral et divers caractères morphologiques du crâne ou des membres, à un état relativement peu éloignée du stade anthropoïde. Il n'est pas exagéré de considérer des telles appréciations comme résultant d'un préjugé et même d'un préjugé irrité, car elles n'étaient pas émises avec la circonspection que leurs auteurs eux-mêmes eussent considérée comme nécessaire en toute autre question.[20]

[Theologians once asked themselves whether women have souls. A few hundred years later, scientists came very close to denying them human intelligence. One can read, in the most prestigious collections of scientific writings, many discussions and conclusions arguing that, in the evolution of the human species, women apparently remain, in many important respects – for example in their cerebral development or various morphological characteristics of the skull or limbs – in a state very little further advanced than anthropoid apes. It is no exaggeration to suggest that such judgements are the result of prejudice, indeed of simple irritation, for they show none of the scholarly consideration that their authors would have deemed essential in relation to any other question.]

In spite of the fact that women in France were becoming educated in ever greater numbers, at the time Pascal qualified as a psychiatrist, the law decreed that if they married, they reverted to the status of minors and could not exercise the functions that, for example, a clinical psychiatrist would be expected to carry out. In a country where women had few civil rights, there was enormous significance in granting women authority in the psychiatric service, one of the major public institutions of the Third Republic. Pascal's response to this paradox was pragmatic. She was certainly aware of male prejudice within the scientific community, so she used her authority, wit and charm to combat it. If all her male colleagues were not feminists, the meritocracy of the examination system did allow women to succeed. In her own lifetime, however, marriage remained an unlikely possibility to be combined with a woman's professional life.

Though Constance Pascal stands out as a 'first' in the hitherto all-male psychiatric profession, the lower echelons of psychiatric

20 Léonce Manouvrier, 'Conclusions générales sur l'anthropologie des sexes et ses applications sociales' [General conclusions on sexual anthropology and its social applications], *Revue de l'École d'Anthropologie de Paris*, 13 (1903), 405–23.

hospitals were in fact staffed by an army of nurses, most of them female. Their work was extremely onerous, often dealing with highly disturbed patients in conditions of minimal hygiene. It was also dangerous – the murder or injury of staff by deranged patients was by no means uncommon. These women, poorly paid and poorly trained, were, professionally speaking, almost invisible, a fact that may have made their employment in 'unfeminine work' acceptable. The genteel shibboleths about female frailty and decorum surrounding the professional employment of women as doctors, lawyers or journalists did not extend to the employment of the working class. An analysis of nursing staff at the Asylum of Maison Blanche between 1900 and 1910, for example, reveals that 62% had no nursing diploma and some 80% were under thirty years old.[21] Their average length of service was short, a reflection, no doubt, of unpalatable working conditions and poor pay. Pascal was keenly aware of the crucial role played by nursing staff and the dangers they faced. She notes in her annual report of 1932 at Maison Blanche that there was only one night nurse for eighty-five patients: 'En cas de menace de la part d'une aliénée devenue subitement dangereuse, elle est exposée à la mort'[22] [In the event of an attack from a patient who has suddenly become dangerous, she could be killed]. In 1933 she reports: 'C'est grâce au dévouement remarquable de mes infirmières que mon service encombré a fonctionné d'une façon normale. C'est grâce à elles que j'ai pu traiter avec succès les aliénées susceptibles de guérison' [It is thanks to the remarkable devotion of our nurses that my overcrowded clinic has functioned normally. It is thanks to them that I have succeeded in treating the patients capable of being cured].[23] Pascal also gave courses for the nurses in her hospitals, a novelty at a time when psychiatric nurses had almost no training.

Born in 1877 in Pitesti, a medium-sized town north-west of Bucharest in the province of Walachia, Constance Pascal was the daughter of landed gentry. Walachia, where her family owned several agricultural estates, was a fertile farming region. An arresting description of the town and region by her nephew Ion, written in 1938, offers a glimpse of a rural, peasant world untouched by

21 Roger Métivier, 'Les infirmières du début du siècle aux années 30' [Nurses from the beginning of the century to 1930], *Maison Blanche: le centenaire, 1900–2000* (Actes de la journée du Centenaire de Maison Blanche, 22 juin 2000), 51–2.

22 Asile de Maison Blanche, *Rapport* de Mlle le Dr Pascal, Médecin, Chef de la 1re section (1932), 174.

23 Asile de Maison Blanche, *Rapport* de Mlle le Dr Pascal (1933), 160 and Métivier, 'Les infirmières', 58.

industrialization, and the place of the Pascal family in Romanian society:

> Pitesti est une très petite ville de province à environ 100 kilomètres de Bucarest. Située dans une région de hautes collines sous le massif des Carpates de Valachie, elle est peut-être l'une des plus jolies villes de province de chez nous. C'est de là que partirent au 13ᵉ siècle les premiers princes valaques qui conquéraient bientôt toute la région comprise entre le Danube, les Carpates et la Mer Noire et fonderaient ainsi la première principauté roumaine. C'est [*de*] là que venaient nos ancêtres – braves gens cultivant en dilettantes leurs propriétés et dépensant toujours plus que leur revenu. C'est d'ailleurs ce que faisaient tous les grands propriétaires chez nous, qui, vers la fin du dernier siècle, venaient dépenser leur fortune à Paris ou sur le Côte d'Azur. Nos grands-parents n'eurent bientôt plus rien à dépenser et moururent presque pauvres.[24]
>
> [Pitesti is a very small provincial town about 100 kilometres from Bucharest. Situated in a region of high hills, under the Carpathian massif of Walachia, it is perhaps one of the prettiest provincial towns we have. This is where the first Wallachian princes left from, later, to conquer the region between the Danube, the Carpathians and the Black Sea and thus found the first Romanian principality. And our ancestors – fine folk – were also from here, cultivating their lands in an amateurish way and always spending more than they made. Actually that is what all our great landowners did, and towards the end of the last century they would go and spend their fortunes in Paris or on the Côte d'Azur. Our grandparents soon had nothing more to spend and died virtually penniless.]

The Romania of Pascal's childhood was still a feudal society, based on a peasant economy with often-absentee landlords and rigid class divisions. Ion Pascal offers a romantic appreciation of this pre-industrial world: 'C'est un des plus beaux pays d'Europe et cela parce qu'il est resté à l'état nature [*sic*]. La civilisation n'a pas encore fait son œuvre. C'est le seul pays où l'on puisse rêver librement, où les villages sont encore des villages et où la campagne garde encore toute sa poésie' (Corr JP & JP, PRFP, 1 June 1938) [It is one of the most beautiful countries in Europe and that is because it has remained in a state of nature. Civilization has not yet left a mark on it. It is the only country where one can dream freely, where the villages are still villages and the countryside still retains all its poetry].

24 Correspondance Jean Pascal & Jeanne Pascal, Berlin, PRFP (13 May 1938).

Writing over one hundred years earlier, in 1820, the British Consul reports a similarly untouched world but detects behind it a much darker reality:

> There does not perhaps exist a people labouring under a greater degree of oppression from the effect of despotic power and more heavily burdened with impositions and taxes than the peasants of Wallachia and Moldavia, nor any who would bear half their weight with the same patience and seeming resignation.[25]

This 'seeming resignation' eventually evaporated in the peasants' revolt of 1907. Savagely repressed by the authorities, the rebellion reflected hunger for land and resentment against the *rentier* class. The peasants had no share in the prosperity the country had experienced. 'Thanks to the peasants' work, the country can export six times as much grain today, yet the peasant has in no way profited by his work and productivity: on the contrary, his condition is increasingly miserable.'[26]

Although, in 1877, Romania had become an independent state with all the trappings of party representation, this failed to produce genuine pluralism. The political class that emerged was cut off from the peasant base of the country. The boyars, or landlords, dominated the political class. Their sons were sent to be educated abroad, further isolating them from their own culture. This was the career pattern followed by Trajan, Constance Pascal's elder brother, who was educated in the army officer corps in Berlin. Unsurprisingly, deep divisions persisted in the army between the educated classes, trained abroad, and the soldiers from peasant backgrounds, whose way of life and poverty made them an enigma to their superiors. This elitism of class and culture left its mark too on Pascal, in the social assurance she projected. Though she felt her sex was a handicap in terms of her ambitions, the sense of belonging to a superior intellectual and social elite was a strong element in her character. Yet, for this highly intelligent and ambitious young woman, the Romania of her childhood constituted a stifling atmosphere.

Turning from their stagnant political life, Romanian intellectuals looked to Western Europe, and especially France, for cultural inspiration. The existence of a strong francophone culture in Romania meant that French language, literature and social habits were the universal currency of the landed and educated classes.

25 Robert William Seton-Watson, *A History of the Romanians from Roman Times to the Completion of Unity* (Cambridge: Cambridge University Press, 1934), 219.

26 Constantine Stere quoted in R. W. Seton-Watson, 386.

Little is known of Pascal's primary and secondary education except that she studied for the baccalaureate in Bucharest. Because in later years she quarrelled with her Romanian family, she seems to have suppressed accounts of her childhood. She passed on no anecdotes of her early life to her daughter. What is clear is that along with the French language Pascal absorbed the ethos and aspirations of Republican France. When she went to Paris in 1897 at the age of twenty, she had already received a thoroughly French linguistic and cultural orientation. Her determination to achieve a sound academic education, which she equated with French culture, demonstrates not only her intellectual powers, but also her yearning for wider horizons: 'J'avais soif d'instruction' [I was thirsty for knowledge].[27]

Constance Pascal's relations with her Romanian family were complex and tortuous. Her profound sense of anger and injustice concerning her treatment as a girl in relation to her more fortunate brother, who was encouraged in his studies and his military career, was a driving force. Pascal rarely spoke of her family to her daughter and this deliberate and prolonged rupture concealed a lifelong trauma. As she wrote in an undated letter to her sister-in-law, Marie Pascal: 'Décidément la famille, le sentiment de la famille est bien compliqué et je comprends les aliénés qui le perdent' [Decidedly the family, or family feeling, is very complicated and I can understand how mad patients may lose it altogether].[28]

Pascal's ambition to study abroad and to gain further professional qualifications was opposed by her father. After all, well brought-up young ladies in Romania did not envisage professional or intellectual goals. They were expected to marry and carry on the family line. All we know of Pascal's opinion of her father emerges in a terse comment to Trajan: 'Mon père ne voulait pas que j'étudie et disait qu'il fallait t'instruire seulement toi' (Corr CP & TP, PRFP, 28 May 1912 or 13) [My father did not want me to study and said only *you* needed an education]. Her father's death brought liberation, in that the wider Pascal family, comprising her mother and numerous aunts and uncles, allowed her to continue her studies, first in Romania and then in France, though with minimal support. Writing to her brother in defence of her scholastic ambitions, Pascal outlines her academic struggles:

27 Correspondence Constance Pascal & Trajan Pascal, at Clermont Fitz-James, PRFP (undated 1910–13).

28 Correspondence Constance Pascal & Marie Pascal, PRFP (undated 1910–13).

> J'ai passé mon baccalauréat à 17 ans à force de faire toujours deux classes en une année. J'ai voulu continuer; tu te rappelles les difficultés qu'il y a eues [*sic*] lorsque j'ai dit que je voulais faire de la médicine. Ma tante m'a mise à la porte; la pauvre dirigeait mal sa barque [...] elle ne pouvait pas m'aider.[29] Pour faire mes études, je suis rentrée chez M. Va.[30] J'ai enseigné la minéralogie et la chimie; j'ai gagné mon pain pendant deux ans. A 20 ans, le Conseil de Famille a décidé qu'il fallait faire mes études à Paris (Corr CP & TP, PRFP: undated 1912–13).

> [I sat my baccalaureate at seventeen by taking two courses in one year. I wanted to continue; you remember what difficulties there were when I said that I wanted to study medicine. My aunt sent me away; the poor woman was finding it hard to manage; she could not help me. To carry on with my studies I went back to M. Va's school where I taught mineralogy and chemistry, and earned my own living for two years. When I was twenty, the Family Council decided I should study in Paris.]

Pascal seems to have been very attached to her mother, who remained a powerful emotional link, and felt guilty at leaving her behind in Romania: 'Je ne la vois pas mais je sens son coeur de mère qui veille sur moi de loin. C'est comme un sentiment de sécurité dans ma vie solitaire et pleine de soucis' [I can't see her, but I sense her mother's heart watching over me from afar. It is like a feeling of security in my life here which is lonely and full of cares] (Corr CP & MP, PRFP, *c.* 1912–13). She attempted to justify her neglect, while recognising that Mme Pascal had felt abandoned:

> J'ai quitté ma mère pour m'instruire et pour gagner mon pain. [...] Je n'ai pas donné à ma mère l'affection qu'elle méritait. Je me le reproche et je verse des larmes amères. Mais lorsqu'il faut gagner le pain quotidien, le sentiment filial le plus fort se laisse dominer par la lutte pour la vie. Elle l'avait compris. Ses lettres avaient établi entre nous une grand intimité de cœur; elle savait que je luttais avec la vie et que je ne pouvais lui donner que ce que mes devoirs me permettaient (Corr CP & TP, PRFP, 28 May 1912–13).

> [I left my mother in order to get an education and support myself. [...] I did not give my mother the affection she deserved. I feel bad about this and shed bitter tears. But when one is forced to earn one's daily bread, the strongest daughterly feeling must give way to the struggle for life. She understood this. Her letters created a great sense

29 This may be her Aunt Mitte, who is referred to later in having a child late in life. She seems to have given Pascal support for a time, perhaps when she was studying in Bucharest.

30 Name as given in letter, possibly an abbreviation.

> of closeness between us; she knew I was struggling with life and could only offer her what was left after I had fulfilled my obligations.]

According to Constance, Mme Pascal seems to have been dominated by her husband and later by her son Trajan who, Pascal says, terrorized her. 'Ma mère vivait sous la terreur, ses lettres en font foi. Tu lui prenais tout' [My mother lived in a state of terror, her letters prove it. You robbed her of everything] (Corr CP & TP, PRFP 12 April 1913). From the evidence of Pascal's letters, Trajan, like his father before him, acted out the role of the traditional boyar patriarch.

Though the Pascal family owned land, money does not seem to have been plentiful and according to Ion's letter the family had traditionally spent more than they earned. Constance and Trajan, both academically gifted, needed scholarships to pursue their studies. From an early age Constance felt a sense of horror at the traditional matrimonial expectations confronting her. To Trajan, who had complained about the money devoted to her education, she inveighed against the way that young girls of good family were brought up in Romania:

> Quels sont les devoirs des parents envers leurs filles? Pourquoi celles-ci ne font que les classes primaires? On les nourrit jusqu'à leur mariage, sans leur reprocher cette nourriture. On les habille en poupée pour aller au bal et faire la chasse au mari, sans leur reprocher les toilettes et les frais de réception. On les marie; on leur donne une dot et les parents sont heureux de donner leur fille et leur argent. Mon grand tort a été d'avoir fait des études. Dans ma famille arriérée, mon instruction a été une parure inutile qui a coûté cher. Si j'étais restée auprès de ma mère et si je m'étais mariée avec un officier de cavalerie, on aurait dépensé le triple et jamais tu ne me l'aurais reproché. Tu vis au Moyen Age (Corr CP & TP, PRFP *c.*1912–13).

> [What are the duties of parents towards their daughters? Why do girls study no further than primary school? They are given board and lodging until they marry, and no one blames them for the food they eat. They are dressed up like dolls to go to balls and hunt for husbands, and no one blames them for the money spent on clothes or the cost of attending functions. They are married off, given a dowry and their parents are happy to give away their daughters and their money. My great crime was to study. In my backward family, my education was considered a useless and costly ornament. If I had stayed with my mother and married a cavalry officer, the family would have spent three times the sum and you would never have blamed me for it. You are living in the Middle Ages.]

Pascal's rage and sense of injustice against her 'backward' family fuelled her determination to succeed professionally. In comparing her upbringing and her struggle to educate herself with her brother's education, the same letter is enlightening as to the sources of her feminism:

> Tu comprends comment j'ai travaillé, combien j'ai eu de la peine à gagner mon pain dans un pays étranger, moi, femme seule, sans aucune relation, ou sans autre chose que mon travail. Toi, intelligent, tu parles, tu te vantes de gagner ton pain depuis l'âge de seize ans. Sens-tu le ridicule de cet orgueil puéril? Sens-tu combien tu fais peu preuve d'observation sociologique? As-tu jeté un coup d'œil sur la société: n'as-tu pas vu que toutes les écoles, toutes les fonctions sont largement ouvertes aux hommes seulement (surtout il y a vingt ans) [...] n'importe quel imbécile du sexe masculin, qui sait un peu lire et écrire, peut entrer dans une école de l'État? Quel mérite d'être un homme!
>
> [You know how I worked, how difficult it was for me to earn my living in a foreign country, I, a single woman, without any connections, with only my work to sustain me. You, who are intelligent, you talk – boast – about having earned your living since the age of sixteen. Don't you understand how ridiculous this childish pride is? Don't you realize that this just shows how little you know of how the world works? Have you ever taken a look at society? Haven't you noticed that every school and all professional posts are wide open to men only (especially twenty years ago) [...] any idiot of the male sex who can read and write a little can go to a state school. What is the great merit in being a man?]

Pascal's remarkable intellectual drive and ambition sustained her during her struggles to qualify for the baccalaureate in Romania and then in 1897 to begin medical studies in Paris with little and sometimes no money from her family. This period left an indelible impression. She was not above evoking the terror of those difficult years to draw on Trajan's sympathy. Her sense of insecurity and abandonment was still fresh in 1913 when she was already a fully qualified psychiatrist. She reminded Trajan that family income had been set aside for their education and that while at the beginning of her Paris studies she received 250 francs per month, this sum had eventually ceased:

> Tu as vu comment on me laissait mourir de faim, que je suis restée trois mois, [...] sans le sou dans Paris et sans l'aide de mes amies, il

> ne me restait qu'à mourir, me jeter dans la Seine. Travailler comme je l'ai fait, souffrir la faim, le froid, ne recevant pas le minimum de l'assistance et devoir entendre qu'on s'est sacrifié pour moi! (Corr CP & TP, PRFP, 12 August 1913).
>
> [You saw how they left me to die of hunger: for three months [...] I was in Paris without a penny of support and if it hadn't been for the help of my friends, I would have had no choice but to throw myself in the Seine. To work as I did, to suffer from hunger and cold, receiving not the slightest help, and then to be told that you all sacrificed yourself for me!]

Admittedly she writes of these privations in the light of an intense quarrel with her brother concerning their shared inheritance. Her will, drawn up in 1918, makes mention of a property in Romania to be sold in the event of her death.[31] This and other properties may have been disputed by Trajan. But it was not only the lack of money that was a source of grief. Her brother, she felt, did not understand either what she had suffered or what she had achieved.

Her mother's death, in December 1912 or early 1913, threw Pascal into a period of prolonged depression. She complained of physical prostration and was sure she would soon die. She did not return to Romania for her mother's funeral and justified her absence on a number of grounds – her ill health, her overwhelming grief, and the fact that in any case she would have arrived too late. Her explanations, anguished and contradictory, show her mired in misery and guilt:

> C'est fini; ma mère morte, ma vie n'a plus d'attaches. Lorsque tu m'as envoyé le télégramme, j'ai eu subitement les jambes coupées, j'ai senti le malheur. Je n'ai pas pu trouver la force pour partir. [...] Partie je serais arrivée vendredi, le lendemain de l'enterrement. Trop tard, je serais tombée sur sa tombe fraîche. J'agonise comme une malheureuse dans mon lit. Ah! quel malheur pour moi. Si tu savais comme ses lettres étaient bonnes et le bien qu'elles m'ont fait. Toi, tu as ton enfant, ta femme. Moi je n'ai que son souvenir (Corr CP & TP, PRFP, *c.*1913).
>
> [It's all over; with my mother dead I have no more attachments. When you sent me the telegram, my legs turned to water; I felt true misery. I just didn't have the strength to leave. [...] If I had, I would have arrived on Friday, the day after the funeral: too late, I would have collapsed on her freshly dug grave. I lie in my bed, miserable

31 Constance Pascal, 'Mon Testament', PRFP (16 March 1918).

> and near death myself. What misery this is to me. If you knew how good her letters were and what good they did me. You have your child and your wife. I have nothing but her memory.]

Pascal's grief turned to despair and rage on receiving letters from Trajan claiming that her expenses as a student meant that she should not share equally in their joint inheritance. All the bitterness of those years, when she felt herself slighted by him and her family, reappears with redoubled force. When he accuses her of wasting a share of the family's assets on her education, she replies: 'Tu as été mon plus grand ennemi. Tu m'as fait le plus grand mal, à moi, ta sœur, par ton égoïsme, par ton indifférence, par ton désir inassouvi de t'enrichir' [You have been my worst enemy. You have done me the greatest harm – to me, your sister – by your egotism, your indifference, and your insatiable desire for riches]. She further accuses him of terrifying their mother: 'Elle est morte maintenant. Elle ne tremblera plus devant toi. Moi, je n'ai pas peur de tes vociférations; tu peux crier, je te dirai la Vérité. Ma mère vivait dans la terreur, ses lettres en font foi. Tu lui prenais tout; le capital, tout a été à toi' [She is dead now. She will no longer tremble before you. I am not afraid of your shouting and accusations, I will tell you the Truth. My mother lived in terror; her letters prove it. You took everything from her; her capital, everything went to you] (Corr CP & TP, PRFP, *c.* 1913). This correspondence, anguished, intemperate and drawing heavily on self-pity as well as anger, was kept by Trajan and eventually passed to Pascal's daughter, suggesting that he too could not forget their sibling rivalries and quarrels.

In spite of the emotional testimony of these letters, all was not loneliness and penury for this Romanian student in *Belle Époque* Paris. She moved in intellectual circles, making the acquaintance, among others, of the novelist Romain Rolland, the socialist politician Jean Jaurès, who at the time was engaged in campaigning for Dreyfus's exoneration, and Paul Strauss, a radical journalist, senator and social reformer.[32] The highly charged family conflicts do not appear in the public face that Pascal successfully projected here. Among her Parisian friends she exuded confidence and charm. This persona was reflected in an article in a fashionable woman's magazine, lauding Constance, in particular, after she and Madeleine Pelletier passed the examination for Intern of Asylums in 1903. It is a revealing example of a reporter's attempts

32 Rees, 'ÀPCP', 175.

to reconcile female academic merit with traditional femininity. Though mentioning Madeleine Pelletier, already notorious for her brusque manner, short hair and mannish clothes, whose campaign it was that resulted in the examination for interns in the asylums being opened up to women, the writer became openly enthusiastic on the subject of Mlle Pascal:

> Un autre médecin, Mlle Pascal, appartient aujourd'hui à l'asile de Vaucluse. Celle-ci est étrangère, comme beaucoup de femmes médecins: elle est roumaine. 'Ses grands yeux noirs', écrivait, non sans lyrisme, un journaliste en 1904, 'rappellent son pays. Sa manière de parler ferme et précise indique une dose d'énergie dont elle a toujours fait preuve. Son extérieur est fort agréable; elle est toujours vêtue de noir qui lui sied à merveille. Quant à sa coiffure, un chignon fait avec soin et deux bandeaux bien arrangés nous prouvent qu'une certaine coquetterie et l'esthétique physique ne sont pas incompatibles avec la science.' Et il est piquant de voir cette jeune femme, qui compte déjà parmi les savants, tenir la science pour une sainte et grande chose, et aussi pour une parure de plus.[33]

> [Another doctor, Mlle Pascal, has now been posted to the Vaucluse Asylum. She is a foreigner, like many women doctors – a Romanian. One journalist wrote lyrically in 1904: 'Her large dark eyes call to mind her country of birth. Her firm, precise way of speaking suggests the reserves of energy that she has always shown. Her appearance is most pleasing: she always dresses in black, which suits her wonderfully. As for her hair, a carefully arranged chignon and two neat plaits show that a certain coquetry and aesthetic sense are not incompatible with learning'. And there is a piquancy in seeing this young woman, who is already counted among the learned, hold up science as a great and holy ideal, and as a further adornment to her person.]

Profiling eight women doctors, the anonymous author stresses their feminine and maternal qualities. The majority were married, a fact that reassured the journalist about the propriety of their undertaking medical studies. Madeleine Pelletier, who could not be passed over because of her public campaign, and Constance Pascal, who was also single, were potentially more problematic. Pelletier could scarcely provide comfort to anyone looking to reconcile

33 Anon, 'Femmes internes, hôpitaux et asiles', *La Vie heureuse* (February 1905). On the editorial stance of the fashionable *La Vie heureuse*, 'volontiers snob' [deliberately snobbish], see Christophe Charle, *Le Siècle de la Presse, 1830–1939* (Paris: Seuil, 2004), 193.

feminine intellectual potential with domestic ideology. It is with relief that the reporter discovers Pascal's attractive femininity and makes great play with it. He or she would not be the last journalist to do so. Dressed in black, showing an almost nun-like decorum, she conformed to the feminine ideal.

How did Constance herself see her gender position? Did she consider herself to be a feminist? Such a commitment may seem unlikely given her lack of militancy in feminist groups and the journalistic reports, like the one quoted above, which eulogized her femininity.[34] Such a view is almost certainly mistaken. Pascal retained a visceral sense of women's inferior position. She held fiercely to the dignity conferred on her by her abilities and her professional status. She fought for the improvement of nurses' training and conditions of service in the hospitals where she worked. She was proud to have been the first woman to serve as an expert medical/psychiatric witness at courts martial dealing with shell-shock victims; she welcomed during her lifetime the growing number of women seeking psychiatric posts and she brought up her own daughter to be intellectually and financially independent. However, with the exception of one newspaper article that she published in 1919 advocating women's suffrage, she did not take a public stand in the great debates of the day over female emancipation.[35] She certainly did not follow the militant feminism of her colleague, Madeleine Pelletier. Like other ambitious and able women, she strove to prove by her example of professional dedication, rather than by suffragist campaigns, that women could succeed in formerly all-male professions.

Pascal's political caution was partly based on her status as a Romanian national in France. In her early student years in Paris and later as a hospital intern, as a foreigner hoping to gain citizenship, she could not risk public, radical positions. On 2 March 1907, she finally succeeded in gaining naturalization, for which a ten-year period of residence with good behaviour had been required.[36]

34 Sowerwine, 'MP', 1189; Gordon, *IF*, 70–71.

35 Constance Pascal, 'La femme française votera-t-elle?', *La Voix commune* (13 April 1919).

36 A. Adreani, *La Condition des étrangers en France et la législation sur la nationalité française* (Lois des 26 juin, 1889, 22 juillet et 8 août 1893) (Paris: Librairie Guillaumin et Cie, 1896), 112–13. Constance Pascal's naturalization is recorded in the *Bulletin des lois de la République Française, XIIe série, partie supplémentaire,* Tome LXXIV, Bulletin 4137, Paris (2 March 1907), 3379, AVP.

French citizenship was crucial in making her eligible to sit the competitive examination for a permanent psychiatric post in 1908, which she became the first woman to pass successfully. Yet, in spite of a glowing testimonial from the Prefect of the Seine, her candidacy for the *concours* had not-been straightforward, even after the bar against women candidates was abolished in 1906.[37] The Ministry of the Interior queried whether as a naturalized citizen, she would be eligible for public employment. The reply from the Ministry of Justice confirmed (albeit negatively), that the law of 26 June 1881 relating to nationality made no restrictions on employment for naturalized citizens.

Pascal was also sensitive about the possible implications of her Romanian origins. Romanian women in France had a reputation for loose morals and at home in Pitesti there were people prepared to suggest that she was simply 'living it up' in Paris. She was at pains to compensate, or perhaps over-compensate, for this generalized reputation and was deeply upset by the effect that malicious gossip had had on her mother. Constance reproached Trajan for not defending her good name at home:

> L'acte d'un vrai frère serait d'aller gifler publiquement ce calomniateur, malgré qu'il ait été le cousin de sa femme. Pour moi, ces calomnies ne me touchent guère. Ma vie a été au grand jour; j'ai toujours vécu dans les grands établissements de l'État, j'ai travaillé continuellement; j'ai remporté des succès qu'une femme qui a envie de s'amuser ne peut faire. Je tourne le dos à ces êtres bas qui ne m'arrivent pas à mon petit doigt, mais j'ai souffert lorsqu'on me l'a dit à cause des larmes de ma mère. Toi, officier roumain, tu avais à défendre mon honneur, celui de ta famille, le tien même. Tu ne l'as pas fait (Corr CP & TP, PRFP, *c.*1913) (Pascal's emphasis).

> [A true brother would have called this slanderer out in public and struck him, even if he was your wife's cousin. As for me, slanders scarcely affect me. My life is an open book; I have spent it in the great establishments of the state; I have worked ceaselessly and I have achieved successes which a woman who just wanted to amuse herself would never have achieved. I have no time for people like that, who are not worthy to lick my boots, but I did suffer when I was told about it, because of my mother's pain. You, a Romanian officer, should have defended my honour, the honour of your family and indeed your own. You did nothing.]

37 Prefect of the Seine to Minister of Justice, DCPCAC (11 January 1908).

Constance Pascal's decision to specialize in psychiatry over medicine as a career was both a choice and a necessity. Psychiatry was a state-funded profession and financially secure. Psychiatric hospital interns and doctors were sure of a salary.[38] To go into general medicine, which was not state-supported, required private means. As Pascal said of this decision: 'A 25 ans j'ai passé l'Internat des Asiles; j'ai quitté les hôpitaux parce que pour être interne des hôpitaux il faut être riche, on n'est pas payé. Dans les asiles, j'avais mon pain' [At twenty-five I sat the exam for interns in the asylum system, I left the hospital system because in order to be an intern in general medicine one must be rich; there is no pay. In the asylums, I had enough to live on] (Corr CP & TP, PRFP, *c.* 1913). The economic imperative was by no means the only reason for choosing psychiatry. Fundamentally she was fascinated by mental medicine and felt an enduring concern for her patients' disorders.

Pascal's period as an intern, first at Perray Vaucluse under Drs Dupain and Vigouroux and then at Ville Evrard under Dr Paul Sérieux, resulted in the resounding success of her thesis, *Formes atypiqes de la paralysie générale* [Atypical forms of general paralysis] (1905), supervised by Sérieux.[39] He remained a loyal friend and supporter throughout Pascal's career, acting as her referee when she sought changes in asylum postings. His report on her at Ville Evrard read: 'Elle occupe les fonctions d'interne à l'entière satisfaction de ses chefs de service' [She carries out the role of hospital intern to the entire satisfaction of her superiors] (DCPCAC 18 December 1907). General paralysis, in which Pascal had specialized, and which was thought to be a degenerative disease, was in fact identified in 1905 by Shaudin and Hoffmann, who discovered Treponema pallidum in syphilitic patients, as being not a distinct disease but a tertiary stage of syphilis. The year 1906 saw the development of the Wassermann test, which allowed for early diagnosis and some prevention of transmission, though not cure. The French psychiatric establishment was initially reluctant to make the link between syphilis and general paralysis (which in its later stages

38 For the development of psychiatry and psychiatric hospitals in France see Jan Goldstein, *Console and Classify: The French Psychiatric Profession in the Nineteenth Century* (Cambridge: Cambridge University Press, 1987), 276–307.

39 Barbier, *VOCP*, 26–7 and 60–9. For Paul Sérieux see Edward Shorter, *Historical dictionary of Psychiatry* (Oxford: Oxford University Press, 2005), 267–79. Dr Vigouroux was President of the Société Médico-Psychologique from 1914 to 1916.

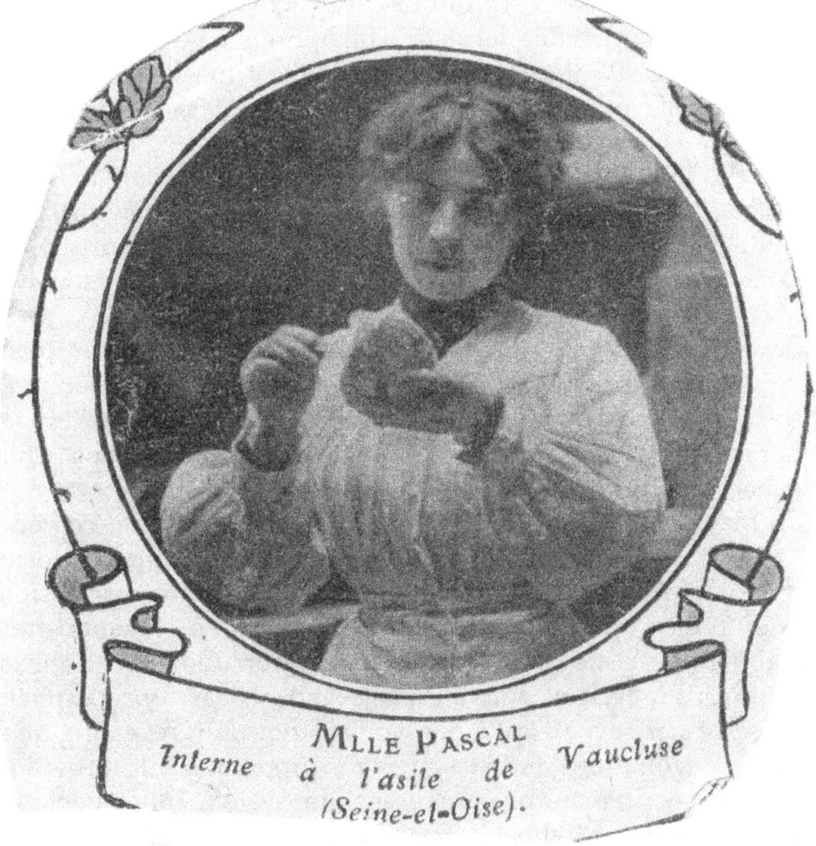

Fig 1. Constance Pascal as an intern at the Vaucluse Asylum

included dementia).[40] Completing her study of atypical forms of general paralysis in 1905, Pascal found herself working at the end, rather than the beginning, of a diagnostic tradition, which helps to explain her subsequent shift in research activity to *démence précoce* [*dementia praecox*], later termed schizophrenia by Eugen Bleuler in 1911. Her 1905 thesis gained the highest mark of *très bien,* a bronze medal from the medical faculty and, in 1906, the prestigious Moreau de Tours prize.[41] Thereafter, Pascal redirected her research, under the influence of Sérieux, who supported Emile Kraepelin's theories on *dementia praecox,* co-authoring an article with Joseph Rogues de Fursac on the subject in 1908. Rogues de Fursac, who became *médecin chef* at Ville Evrard in 1913, published a statistical study on the heredity of patients suffering from general paralysis. He was a proponent of theories of inherited causes of insanity and an advocate of degeneration theory. Although Pascal collaborated with him in one article, she would become increasingly resistant in her subsequent publications to the fatalistic assumptions behind degeneration theory.[42]

In the course of her career from 1908 to 1937, Pascal served in six psychiatric hospitals, first as *médecin adjoint* [junior doctor] and then as *médecin chef* [consultant]. Her cumulative professional dossier in the *Centre d'Archives Contemporaines* (CAC) demonstrates the difficulties she faced in seeking promotion or transfers, sometimes for lack of suitable posts and at least once explicitly because of her sex. Pascal's dossiers are not only revealing about her own negotiations and struggles for promotion but throw light on employment patterns in the asylum system more generally. For any candidate who had passed the qualifying examination in psychiatry, an appropriate post might not be available or the candidate might not wish to take up the post offered. Over the years Pascal and her supporters bombarded the Section of Social Welfare and Public Hygiene of the Ministry of the Interior, which was the central ministry responsible for the psychiatric service, with myriad requests, often to the extreme annoyance of civil servants. Her many disputes with asylum directors, who headed the administrative branch of the hospital, separate from the medical

40 For the acceptance of the Wassermann test for syphilis in France see Claude Quétel, *History of Syphilis* (Oxford: Oxford University Press, 1992).

41 Barbier, *VOCP*, 26–27.

42 Joseph Rogues de Fursac et Constance Pascal, 'Adipose douloureuse chez un dément précoce' [Painful fatty deposits in a *dementia praecox* patient].

hierarchy, became a feature of her official profile. She saw her role as championing the welfare of her patients and was impatient with, if not contemptuous of directors whose limited budgets made it difficult to improve conditions. When it came to requesting a transfer to another hospital, Pascal did not hesitate to evoke her unhappiness and personal suffering in the most emotional terms. If the authorities were frequently exasperated by these appeals, there was, at the same time, an official recognition of her passionate commitment to her work, as well as admiration for her remarkable and sustained research and psychiatric publications.

Pascal's career choice also links her to important aspects of early French feminism, which can be glimpsed in her acquaintance with Madeleine Pelletier. These two young and ambitious women, who were contemporaries and both interns in psychiatry, illustrate widely differing approaches to advancing the cause of women. Pelletier, of working class origins (her father, a cab driver, had been incapacitated by a stroke and her mother ran a tiny vegetable shop near Les Halles), grew up in great poverty in Paris. She stressed the centrality of her feminist convictions: 'Je puis dire que j'ai toujours été féministe, du moins depuis que j'avais l'âge de comprendre' [I can say that I have always been a feminist, at least since I was old enough to understand] (Gordon: *IF*, 7), she wrote in her autobiography. It was Pelletier who, in 1902–03, with the help of the feminist daily paper *La Fronde*, orchestrated the campaign to give women access to the examination for psychiatric internships. Pascal did not take part in this very public campaign, almost certainly from motives of prudence arising from her foreign status. However, she and Pelletier were interns at Ville Evrard Hospital in the eastern suburbs of Paris at the same period. It is difficult to imagine two more contrasting types. Madeleine Pelletier, short and pugnacious, already advertised her feminist convictions by wearing tailored 'mannish' suits and cutting her hair short. This last was seen as an outrageous gesture in a period when women's long hair, tied back in an elaborate chignon, was a key sign of femininity and decorum. Constance Pascal, by contrast, tall, elegant, with a magnificent mane of beautifully arranged black hair, combined feminine charm with aristocratic authority.

A contemporary male intern at Ville Evrard, Dr Paul Courbon, offers us a glimpse of the two young women, in a passage redolent of the gender expectations of the *Belle Époque*. Looking back on his early training, he recalls Constance Pascal with almost breathless enthusiasm, and reads Madeleine Pelletier correctly, if entirely unsympathetically, as her polar opposite:

> Je dois encore une mention à la phalange féminine, qui occupe un nombre de plus en plus grand de places dans nos rangs. Je ne parlerai que de celles qui furent à sa tête et avec qui je vécus en salle de garde: Constanza Pascal et Madeleine Pelletier; elles étaient de la promotion de 1903. Constanza Pascal, née Roumaine et naturalisée Française, alors dans tout l'éclat de la jeunesse, méritait la double épithète que les historiens du Moyen Age décernèrent à une de ses devancières, professeur à l'école de Salerne: Constanza Calenda, aussi belle que savante. Madeleine Pelletier était née à Paris; hantée par sa théorie de l'égalité absolue des sexes, elle eût repoussé comme une injure la première de ces épithètes, elle s'efforçait, par sa mise et ses manières, de ne donner à personne l'idée de la lui appliquer. Elle eut sa notoriété au temps des suffragettes. J'ignore ce qu'elle est devenue.[43]

> [I should mention the female phalanx that occupies today an ever-greater place in our ranks. I will speak only of those who were the first and with whom I lived in the staff room: Constanza Pascal and Madeleine Pelletier, who were in the first year of women interns. Constanza Pascal, born a Romanian and naturalized French, then in all the splendour of her youth, merited the double epithet that the historian of the Middle Ages gave to one of her predecessors, a professor at the [medical] school of Salerno: Constanza Calenda: 'as beautiful as she was learned'. Madeleine Pelletier was born in Paris; obsessed with her theory of the absolute equality of the sexes, she would have rejected as an insult the first of these epithets; she endeavoured, by her dress and her manners to give no-one the idea of applying it to her. She became notorious in the suffragette period. I have no idea what became of her.]

Neither woman has left any recollections of the other, nor do we know of any subsequent contact between them, though they must have been well acquainted as interns. One can easily imagine that Pelletier would have bridled at Pascal's elegance and class assurance and that Pascal would have found Pelletier's touchiness and feminist militancy unattractive. Yet both held profound feminist convictions while approaching the 'woman question' from different

43 Dr Paul Courbon, unpublished MS courtesy of Dr Jacques Chazaud, PRFP. Courbon also co-authored an article with Pascal, 'Délire des préjudices préséniles' [Frenzy resulting from early senile dementia], *L'Encéphale,* 6 (25 November 1906), 573–78.

perspectives. Pelletier refused to negotiate on women's oppression and lived a principled life combating it in word and deed. For her, women who were willing to play the game of femininity in order to succeed in a male world were what she scornfully termed '*demi-féministes*' [semi-feminists] (Gordon, *IF*, 18). As she wrote in 1909, shortly after failing her qualifying examination in psychiatry:

> Les doctoresses, les avocates, les professeurs femmes, les femmes peintres, sculpteurs, les romancières, etc., qui devraient se faire les ardentes propagandistes des idées féministes à l'extension desquelles elles doivent la situation qu'elles occupent, s'en déclarent au contraire soit entièrement détachées, soit même adversaires. Chacune fait effort pour mettre à part sa condition propre du reste du féminisme, dans sa prétention naïve à être une intelligence transcendante qui aurait franchi tous les obstacles et parce qu'elle manque de courage pour avouer une opinion qui n'a pas encore la majorité.[44]
>
> [Women doctors, lawyers, teachers, painters, sculptors and novelists, etc., who should be ardent campaigners for feminist ideas, to whose diffusion they owe their success, declare, on the contrary, that they are entirely uninterested in or even opposed to them. Each one tries to separate her personal condition from the rest of feminism, with the naïve implication that her transcendental intelligence could have overcome all obstacles by itself and because she lacks the courage to admit to convictions that are not yet espoused by the majority.]

Pelletier may well have been thinking – and I would add unfairly – of her erstwhile colleague at Ville Evrard, Constance Pascal.

An opposing view emerges from Pascal's friend and mentor, Mathilde Salomon, principal of the Collège Sévigné, an ardent republican and educational reformer for women.[45] Congratulating Pascal on being the first woman to pass the *concours* for *médecin adjoint*, Salomon wrote:

> Je suis heureuse de voir votre succès; un succès qui grandira, pour vous d'abord, tant l'affection m'est chère, tant la nature riche, aimante et gracieuse m'a conquise – et pour la cause des femmes ensuite. *Vous êtes féministe comme j'aime que l'on soit: en agissant, non en réclamant.* Comme vous allez mettre tout votre dévouement, votre étonnante

44 Madeleine Pelletier, 'Le féminisme et ses militantes', *Documents du progrès* (July 1909), 20.

45 See Catherine Nicault, 'Mathilde Salomon, pédagogue et pionnière de l'éducation féminine', *Archives juives*, 1: 37 (2004), 129–34.

> activité, votre belle vaillance au service de votre grande œuvre, tout ira admirablement et personne ne vous contestera l'autorité nécessaire, que vos fonctions comportaient et que la nature vous a donnée.[46]
>
> [I am happy to see your success, a success which will increase; happy for you, first of all, so fond as I am of you, so won over as I have been by your generous, affectionate and gracious nature and secondly, happy for the cause of women. You are the kind of feminist I like best: a feminist of action, not of demands. Since you will be putting all your devotion, your amazing energy, your splendid courage to the service of your great work, everything will go splendidly and no-one will begrudge you the authority your profession demands and with which nature has endowed you.]

Mathilde Salomon gave Pascal some teaching to eke out her meagre student income and remained a role model for Pascal as a professional woman. Many years later, in recognition of her debt to Salomon, Pascal enrolled her daughter for her secondary school studies at the Collège Sévigné.

Fiercely ambitious, like Pelletier, and often scornful in private of male pretensions, Pascal was prepared nevertheless to use both her sex and her class to good effect in her profession. Negotiating the male hierarchy of the hospital world was not easy. In the course of her career she had long-drawn-out battles with asylum directors, whom she tended to characterize as examples of male arrogance and embattled correspondence with civil servants at the Ministry of Health. However, the male medical-psychiatric world could be daunting for women. Madeleine Pelletier recalled that she had been harassed by male interns for her mode of dressing and when unsuccessful at her first attempt at the *concours* for *médecin adjoint*, she was barred by age from attempting the examination a second time. She abandoned psychiatry for private medical practice, turning her enormous energy to socialist and feminist militancy.[47] Constance Pascal succeeded in the male professional world, through her abilities and acute intelligence, but also by maintaining a feminine persona. The divergences in life strategies between these two remarkable and talented women – direct confrontation, as

46 Corr Mathilde Salomon & CP, PRFP (4 February 1909), emphasis mine.

47 Candidates were only eligible for the examination for *médecin-adjoint* (junior doctor) up to the age of thirty-one. Pelletier was thirty-one in 1906, so was precluded from sitting a second time. Constance Pascal was thirty-one in 1908 but passed on the first attempt.

opposed to subversion of gender – starkly illuminated the choices for women entering elite professions in early twentieth-century France.

3. 'A Woman's Pity' – Clermont de l'Oise: 1908–20

In 1908, having passed the examination for *médecin adjoint des hôpitaux*, Pascal was assigned to the Asylum of Clermont de l'Oise in the post of junior doctor. Apart from a two-year secondment to the Saint Maurice asylum, near Paris, she remained there until 1920. This introduction to her medical and psychiatric practice in a provincial hospital proved difficult, not to say traumatic, as she lived through the privations of the First World War, close to the battle fields and, in addition, underwent complex personal crises. In Constance Pascal's journals, kept throughout the 1914–18 War, we have an invaluable record of life in an asylum virtually on the front line.

Although she had passed the *concours* in March 1908, Pascal was not appointed to Clermont until October of the same year. In the interim she remained at Ville Evrard under Dr Paul Sérieux. Negotiations to find a suitable post were prolonged. In July, writing to the Minister of the Interior on Pascal's behalf, a Mme Roussier requested that Pascal be given a post at the Fondation Valet at Bourneville 'pour les jeunes filles incapables de développement' [for girls incapable of normal development] because: 'elle s'intéresse depuis des années spécialement à la question des dégénérées et on peut compter sur la bonté pitoyable dont elle a donné tant de preuves pour veiller au bien-être et au bonheur de ces pauvres petites' [for many years she has been particularly concerned with the question of the mentally handicapped and one may be assured, knowing the compassion of which she has given so many proofs, that she will look after the welfare and wellbeing of these poor little girls].[1] This commendation is the first reference in her dossier relating to Pascal's interest in treating and educating children with severe learning difficulties.

1 Mme Roussier to Minister of the Interior, DCPCAC (1 July 1908). The term 'dégénéré' was applied to the mentally handicapped or simply to those with mental illnesses thought to have an hereditary basis.

The post at Clermont (confirmed on 29 October 1908) gave Pascal a salary of 3,000 francs per annum, with lodging within the hospital, heating and lighting.[2] At the same period, an agricultural worker would earn 28 francs a month or 336 francs a year. Pascal wrote to a friend at the Ministry of the Interior, possibly Georges Clemenceau, thanking him for his efforts on her behalf and expressing enthusiasm for her new post: 'Je sais que c'est à vous que je dois cette joie. Je suis émue de l'intérêt que vous me portez' [I know that I owe this happiness to you. I am touched by the concern you have shown me].[3] Early reports on Pascal from the Prefect were favourable: 'Mlle Pascal est très dévouée à ses fonctions' [Mlle Pascal is very devoted to her work].[4] In 1911 she was promoted to the second grade of her pay scale with a salary of 3,500 francs. This was probably the high point of her career at Clermont.

As the first woman in psychiatry, Pascal was and remained newsworthy throughout her career. Press reports commented on her commitment to reforming asylum practice, especially the abolition of routine punishments and the use of straitjackets. Her humane concern for her patients was entirely genuine, reflecting debates in the media and the psychiatric profession about the care of the insane.[5] The reformers' criticisms had two major facets. The first was a critique of the law of 1838, which established public asylums and laid out the legal framework for the involuntary detention of patients.[6] Concern about the potential for arbitrary imprisonment, the power of doctors to keep patients in asylums, combined with scepticism about the accuracy of psychiatric diagnoses and the efficacy of treatment created an early anti-psychiatry movement. In spite of repeated efforts to modify or reform the law of 1838, no significant legislative changes took place during Pascal's lifetime. In 1924, Pascal was to defend the law of 1838 in an article entitled 'Les Asiles d'aliénés ne sont pas des geôles' [Insane asylums are not jails], arguing that the provisions of the law provided sufficient safeguards for individual

2 Corr Minister of the Interior & Prefect of l'Oise, DCPCAC (29 October 1908).

3 Corr CP & Ministry of the Interior, DCPCAC (17 November 1908).

4 Corr Minister of the Interior & Prefect of l'Oise, DCPCAC (13 December 1909).

5 Ian R. Dowbiggin, *Inheriting Madness: Professionalization and Psychiatric Knowledge in Nineteenth-Century France* (Berkeley: University of California Press, 1991), pp. 93–108.

6 Robert Castel, *L'Ordre psychiatrique: l'âge d'or de l'aliénisme* (Paris: Éditions Minuit, 1976).

liberty. On this issue, she backed the profession's authority against the reformers on the left of the political spectrum.[7]

The second criticism of asylums was the issue of the treatment of patients within the institution. Since Pinel,[8] the idea of moral treatment, aimed at restoring patients to rationality by kindness and good treatment, had, in theory, been the underlying ethos of asylum care. In practice, the huge numbers of patients, over-crowding, minimal sanitation, coupled with poorly trained and badly paid nursing staff meant that the function of many large hospitals was simply to contain their patients. Aggression by and towards patients was common. Violence against inmates fell into two categories: first, as an integral part of their treatment – cold showers, straitjackets, locked caged beds for sleeping – all supposedly to protect patients from harming themselves or others.[9] Second, violence was frequently, if not routinely, meted out to patients by the nursing staff and warders as punishment for allegedly unruly behaviour, as is evidenced by numerous testimonies of former patients.

With regard to violence of treatment, the psychiatric reformers, in seeking to improve the lot of the mentally ill, called for adoption of the English policy of 'no-restraint'. The result of an enquiry published in 1882 by *Les Annales Médico-psychologiques*, the trade journal for psychiatry, suggested that no-restraint was simply a reworking of Pinel's system.[10] The report concluded that while techniques of restraint should be used as a last resort, they were necessary and unavoidable. Conservative in tone, it nevertheless points to the extent to which public anxiety about the treatment and abuse of patients in mental hospitals had obliged the profession to examine its own practice.

7 Constance Pascal, 'Les Asiles d'aliénés ne sont pas des geôles', *Le Matin* (PRFP, 1924).

8 Philippe Pinel (1745–1826) was a French physician who was instrumental in the development of a more humane psychological approach to the custody and care of psychiatric patients; this is referred to today as the moral treatment.

9 For discussions of the treatment of mental patients see Dowbiggin, *Inheriting Madness*; Aude Fauvel, 'Punition, dégénérescence ou malheur? La folie d'André Gill (1840–1885)', *Revue d'histoire du XIXe siècle* (2003), 26–7; Jan Goldstein, *Console and classify: the French Psychiatric Profession in the Nineteenth Century* (Cambridge: Cambridge University Press, 1987); Yannick Ripa, *Women and Madness: the Incarceration of Women in Nineteenth-century France* (Cambridge: Polity Press, 1986).

10 Dr Bécoulet, 'Étude sur le No-Restraint', *Les Annales médico-psychologiques*, 6e série, VII, 4e année (1882), 41–69.

When Pascal was posted to the Asylum of Clermont de l'Oise, she joined a hospital with a more than troubled history. By the end of the nineteenth century, Clermont had become the largest asylum in France. It was privately owned, taking many indigent patients paid for by the state. A notorious scandal that had engulfed Clermont in 1880, twenty-eight years before Pascal's arrival, bears directly on her experiences as *médecin adjoint* from 1908 to 1920. What came to be called l'Affaire Appert had for the first time opened a mental hospital to judicial and press scrutiny.[11] In 1880, the chief warder, Estoret, savagely beat and killed a patient named Appert. Although Estoret secretly buried the body, it was eventually discovered. There followed an unprecedented scandal in which Estoret was condemned to life imprisonment with hard labour. The interest of the case for historians and for a contemporary audience, however, rests on the testimony by staff and patients about the violence habitually meted out in the hospital – testimony which had never before been so clearly elicited from a closed asylum. In the Appert Affair, the full light of the criminal justice system was brought to bear on a previously secret world.

Clermont was fairly typical of the enormous 'museums of madness' of the golden age of French psychiatric hospitals.[12] It would appear that in spite of the Appert Affair, the reform of sanitary facilities and coercive treatment of patients had made little progress by the turn of the century. A highly critical view of the asylum can be gleaned from a former director, Monsieur Plantie, who remained at Clermont for only ten months, resigning on 14 April 1908, just prior to Pascal's appointment. In his exposé, entitled 'Le Bagne des fous' [The Penal Colony of the Mad], he alleged that the institution lacked appropriate facilities, suffered from bad hygiene and had insufficient and poorly paid staff. There were 140 nurses for 1687 patients. In the entire hospital there were only 35 baths and 3 showers for a population of patients of whom many were incontinent. In addition, the increasing number of the criminally insane sent to the hospital created a problem of security, or as he put it 'promiscuity'. Plantie contrasted his ideal of what an asylum should be, namely a refuge for the mentally afflicted, with the reality of Clermont:

11 Aude Fauvel, 'Le crime de Clermont et la remise en cause des asiles en 1880', *Revue d'histoire moderne et contemporaine* (2002), 49–61.

12 See Michel Foucault, *Folie et déraison: histoire de la folie à l'âge classique* (Paris: Plon, 1961); Andrew Scull, *Museums of Madness: The Social Organisation of Insanity in Nineteenth-Century England* (London: Allen Lane, 1979); Roy Porter, *Madness: A Brief History* (Oxford: Oxford University Press, 2002).

> Quand on entre dans cet asile, on éprouve une impression sinistre. Les asiles doivent être riants, donner l'idée d'un lieu de repos, où le malade quel qu'il soit, vient se refaire et séjourner après la catastrophe ou le surmenage qui ont eu raison de sa raison. Celui-ci donne l'impression d'un bagne.[13]
>
> [As soon as one enters this asylum, one is struck by its sinister atmosphere. Asylums should be cheerful, places of tranquillity where the patient, whoever he may be, comes to rest and recuperate after a breakdown or recover from the stresses of work which have destroyed his sanity. This asylum is more like a penal colony.]

Pascal had read Plantie's damning report, as is clear from despairing remarks she made in her war journal when, overwhelmed by the depressive effect of her life in this huge institution, she wrote:

> Il faudrait un volume pour décrire l'organisation de l'Asile de Clermont. On a fait un livre intitulé *Le Bagne des fous* qui indique bien combien l'organisation est bonne; ça s'est passé il y a sept ou huit ans. Mais maintenant c'est le bagne des aliénistes.[14]
>
> [It would take a volume to describe the organization of the Clermont Asylum. Someone has written a book called *The Penal Colony of the Mad* which describes how excellent the organization is. That was seven or eight years ago. Now it's the penal colony of the psychiatrists.]

The patients were organized on a class system, based on the ability to pay. At the base were the indigent patients. Then the third, second and first-class patients paid a sliding scale of charges, plus a supplementary charge if they brought a servant with them. The Fitz-James Section, where Pascal was assigned, was situated apart from the main hospital in its own grounds and took a number of 'superior'-class patients. The asylum farm, where many of the more able patients worked, was situated there. Physical labour was seen as both practical (asylums could be almost self-sufficient in food production) and therapeutic. The war created food shortages, however, and on one occasion Pascal informed the Director that several of her patients had gone on hunger strike in protest at the lack of eggs and milk. This asylum population varied with the seasons. Because it was a rural area, families would often withdraw relatives who were interned but able-bodied during harvest time in order to provide extra hands.

13 Quoted in Claude Tillet, 'Le Centre hospitalier spécialisé de Clermont de l'Oise de 1790 à nos jours', *Mémoires de la société archéologique et historique de Clermont en Beauvaisis*, XXXV (1983), 24.

14 Constance Pascal, War Journal, 1914–18, Cahier I, 7, PRFP. All further references will be to CP WJ.

Fitz-James also had a children's section. Thanks to her experience there, Pascal pursued her interest in educating children with severe learning difficulties, publishing an article in 1913 entitled 'L'Enfance anormale dans les maisons de correction' [Handicapped children in reform schools].[15] By creating what she termed 'hospital schools', she hoped to avoid imprisoning children with psychological difficulties, ideas which she would later put into practice at the Châlons sur Marne Asylum.

As a result of Plantie's whistle-blowing efforts, improvements were already under way at Clermont when Pascal arrived, though many of the projected reforms had to be shelved at the outbreak of the war. The high water-mark of patients (1,687 in 1908) decreased somewhat during the war, owing to high mortality rates. Sanitation continued to be poor. Outbreaks of typhoid were common. The Clermont Council blamed the hospital for the spread of infections that attacked the town. Even at Fitz-James, the supposedly luxurious side of the asylum, sewage and slops left a filthy swamp behind the wards. The septic tanks overflowed and the slaughterhouse threw its offal into the nearby stream, creating a stink in the whole area.[16]

If conditions for the majority of patients were bad, those for the staff were hardly ideal. Nurses and night attendants lived in and often used the same facilities as the patients. For the psychiatrists conditions were much better, but they too lived in the grounds of the hospital and were virtually institutionalized. Pascal had an apartment allocated to her. However, her repeated requests for repairs to falling plaster, redecoration and thin partition walls suggest minimal conditions of comfort. She complained that her books and clothes became mouldy, owing to lack of adequate heating and damp walls. Most oppressive was the surveillance exercised upon asylum staff. As a single woman, she believed with reason that she was spied on.

Nevertheless Pascal succeeded in effecting notable reforms in the hospital. Among them were: forbidding the use of corporal punishment and straitjackets for patients; appointing a woman as head of the nursing staff in charge of handicapped children; and (as noted by the inspectorate), having greatly improved the daily life of the patients. She ensured clean and tidy dormitories, that the children were well-cared for and that their surroundings, including colourful flower borders, were cheerful and less forbidding than previously.[17]

15 Constance Pascal, 'L'Enfance anormale dans les maisons de correction', *Revue philanthropique*, XXXIV (1913–1914), 260–71.

16 See Tillet, *Centre hospitalier*, 26–27.

17 Rees, 'ÀPCP', 177.

Thanks to her Parisian contacts, among them the socialist leader Jean Jaurès and Joseph Lefèvre, later minister of war, both editors of *La Petite République,* Pascal was interviewed for an article which appeared in 1911, 'Une femme médecin d'une asile d'aliénés' [An insane asylum's woman doctor]. It reflects both Pascal's initial success in ameliorating conditions at Clermont and the political impetus for reform. The reporter, looking at the asylum from the perspective of the ordinary public and using the vocabulary of the day to describe patients suffering from mental illness ('degenerates' etc.), eulogizes Pascal for the humane reforms she had brought to the hospital, and for her soothing, feminine qualities. We see here evidence of her impressive presence and her enthusiasm for her work balancing the almost unrelieved picture of unhappiness and frustration that emerges from her journals three years later. Very revealing for the contemporary reader is the reporter's casual but shocking comment that epileptic patients are locked away with the 'mad', though it is recognized that they are sane:

> Là-bas dans l'Oise, au pied d'une petite ville sans grâce, dans la campagne givrée aujourd'hui, on a bâti, voilà quelques années, un asile pour les aliénés et pour les épileptiques plus malheureux que les fous. C'est Fitz-James, dépendance de l'asile de Clermont. Sans doute nous ne songerions pas à le mentionner ici, pas plus que tous ceux qui abondent hélas! dans la région de la Seine, s'il n'était pas le seul en France à être confié à la science médicale d'une femme. Cette femme, l'unique qui ait subi avec succès le concours des médecins d'asiles d'aliénés, vit depuis trois ans, dévouée à la plus ingrate des tâches, dans cette solitude, au milieu de ce peuple de dégénérés et de déments, auquel ses soins apportent un peu de soulagement, et sa présence un peu de joie. Car Mlle Pascal est jeune et belle, et lorsqu'elle passe dans les salles gantée et coiffée, avec l'autorité du geste et du regard, le fou le plus agité rassemble un moment, en cette présence, le faible pouvoir d'inhibition qui lui reste pour retenir les fureurs et les propos ignobles. Tous ces malheureux sentent vaguement sous la sagesse du docteur, la pitié de la femme, et sans comprendre toujours, la remercient de sa bonté. L'un d'eux, un épileptique, me disait: 'Ah! si elle n'était pas là, que deviendrions-nous!' Mlle Pascal a interdit les châtiments, fait supprimer la camisole de force.[18]

> [A few years ago, deep in the Oise valley, below a charmless village, in a landscape covered in frost at this season, an asylum was built to house the insane, as well as epileptics, who are more unfortunate than the mad. Named Fitz-James, it is an outlying section of the Clermont

18 L. M. Compain, 'Une femme médecin d'un asile d'aliénés', *La Petite République* (1911).

> Asylum. Doubtless we would not be describing it here, any more than the many asylums that flourish, alas, in the Seine region, if it were not that this is the only one in France to be entrusted to the medical skill of a woman. This woman, the only one who has passed the competitive examination in mental medicine, has dwelt in this solitary place for the past three years, devoting herself to the most thankless of tasks, living in the midst of a population of degenerate and demented souls to whom her care brings a little relief and her presence a moment of joy. For Mlle Pascal is young and beautiful, and when she passes through the wards, gloved and her hair skilfully arranged, with authority in her gestures and expression, the most agitated patient finds the strength to muster for a moment the weak powers of control remaining to him, to restrain his furies and his foul language. All these unfortunates sense somehow that beneath the medical wisdom of the doctor lies a woman's pity and, without always understanding, they thank her for her goodness. One of them, an epileptic, said to me: 'If she were not here, what would become of us?'. Mlle Pascal has forbidden punishments and abolished straitjackets.]

Making her rounds through the wards, Pascal is shown as calming the patients by her mere presence, a Florence Nightingale for the mad. Not only is she lovely to look at, her gloved hands and careful coiffure suggest an eminently lady-like figure. The reforms she has instituted, abolishing straitjackets and punishment beatings are, for the reporter, the result of her feminine qualities of compassion. The profession of asylum doctor, he argues, far from being unsuitable for a woman, is ideally suited to exploit womanly, maternal characteristics:

> Et je pensais que cette carrière de médecin des asiles d'aliénés qui demande, jointe à une science profonde, une si haute dose de dévouement était de celles où les femmes pourraient être appelées à rendre les plus grands services. Les malades de la doctoresse Pascal ne sont pas pour elle seulement des malades et des sujets d'études, ce sont des êtres qu'elle aime parce que leur détresse mentale l'a émue! Ils ne lui inspirent ni répulsion, ni dédain, mais un attachement fait d'intelligente pitié. [...] Peut-être que si d'autres femmes s'adonnaient, comme le fait Mlle Pascal, au soulagement de ces malheureux, leurs efforts hâteraient la venue de ces milieux, dont la création a été souvent désirée, où le demi-dégénéré pourrait atteindre au développement moral et intellectuel dont il est susceptible, et passer sur cette terre des jours moins chargés de peines. Mettre la science au service de la pitié, n'est-ce pas faire une œuvre féminine entre toutes?

> [And it occurred to me that the career of asylum doctor, which requires both profound knowledge and a high degree of devotion, was one where women could be called to do the greatest service. For *doctoresse* Pascal, her patients are not only objects of study, they are

beings whom she loves because their mental distress has touched her. They inspire in her neither repulsion nor disdain, but affection based on intelligent pity. [...] Perhaps if other women devoted themselves, as Mlle Pascal does, to the relief of these unfortunates, their efforts would hasten the creation of the institutions we have so long hoped for: places where the semi-degenerate could achieve the moral and intellectual development of which they are capable, and live less painful lives here on earth. To put science at the service of pity – is that not the most feminine of acts?]

In the early days at Clermont, before the outbreak of war, Pascal must have hoped for great strides in asylum reform, most of which were eventually frustrated by the administration. Her plans for the future, to create familial colonies for less severely afflicted patients, herald the movement for the return of mental health sufferers to the community which was to become characteristic of psychiatric practice in much of Europe from the 1970s onwards. Quoting Pascal's critique of the present system of asylum care and her schemes for improvement, Compain writes:

Tous les fous, tous les maniaques, tous les épileptiques, ne sont pas des 'sujets d'asile'. Il y en a beaucoup dont la manie est intermittente ou douce, dont les crises sont rares, dont le caractère est déformé, mais dont l'esprit est resté lucide, et tous ceux-là souffrent cruellement de leur situation d'internés. Or si on rend à la société ces êtres à demi-déchus ils n'y peuvent subsister. Ils ont des caprices, des tares qui les rendent impropres au travail régulier. Renvoyés, malheureux ils demandent parfois d'eux-mêmes à revenir à l'asile où, du moins, ils ont le pain assuré. Rentrés, ils souffrent plus encore du contact des aliénés incurables, des épileptiques à crises graves et fréquentes, à caractères plus déformés, des idiots, des gâteux. Point de milieu pour eux entre l'asile qui est une prison et la société à laquelle ils ne peuvent s'adapter. Ce milieu il faudrait le créer. On peut se le représenter sous la forme d'un asile-école, d'une colonie surveillée, d'un village artificiel comme il en existe en Angleterre pour les orphelins, ou mieux encore, d'un placement familial surveillé de très près. L'aliénation s'exaspère au contact de l'aliénation, la vue des crises, provoque les crises; à l'aliéné, à l'épileptique peu atteint, moins dégénéré, il faudrait pour recouvrer la santé relative de l'esprit, le contact d'êtres normaux, et la surveillance médicale lui reste indispensable. Le rendre libre à la société pour laquelle il est un danger est impossible; l'enfermer pêle-mêle, avec des malades plus malades que lui-même, est une cruauté.

[Not all the mad, not all lunatics, not all epileptics should be in asylums. There are many whose mania is intermittent or mild, who have only occasional crises, whose personalities are distorted but whose minds remain lucid, and all of these suffer cruelly as sectioned patients. On the other hand, if they are returned to the community, these vulnerable beings cannot survive. Their peculiarities and defects make them unsuitable for regular work. Unemployed, unhappy, they will sometimes ask to return to the asylum, where at least they know there will always be food on their plate. But once back, they suffer even more from contact with the incurably insane, or with epileptics who have frequent severe fits, or from patients with even more deformed personalities, idiots and the demented. There is no natural home for them, between the asylum, which is a prison, and the community, to which they cannot adapt. We must create that home. It might take the form of an asylum-school, a supervised colony, a purpose-built village, like those one finds in England for communities of orphans; or better still, a closely supervised placement in a family. Madness is aggravated by contact with other mad people; seeing other people's attacks provokes one's own attacks. Those with less severe cases of insanity or epilepsy are more likely to recover a reasonable level of mental health through contact with normal people, though of course they need continued medical supervision. Turning such a patient loose in society, where he might pose a threat, is unthinkable; locking him up cheek by jowl with people who are madder than himself is cruel.]

Although Pascal was promoted to the first class of her civil service grade in January 1913, she had grown increasingly discouraged in her efforts to reform asylum practice, as well as suffering from social isolation in that provincial backwater. She wrote revealingly to the minister:

> Je suis très touchée de votre sympathie. Votre lettre vient m'apporter du courage. Depuis quelque temps je commence à sentir l'influence paralysante de la vie des asiles de province. Mlle Roussier a eu pitié de me voir si malheureuse et elle est allée vous parler de moi sans que je le sache. Lorsque vous m'avez offert ce poste, vous m'avez bien prévenue des difficultés que j'allais rencontrer, mais à ce moment-là j'étais jeune, sans expérience et pleine d'enthousiasme; je croyais que l'amour du travail suffisait pour tout vaincre. Je me suis trompée. Aujourd'hui je me sens écrasée par mon milieu.[19]
>
> [I am very touched by your sympathy. Your letter has given me strength. For some time I have begun to feel the paralysing effect of life in a provincial asylum. Seeing my unhappiness, Mlle Roussier [*her advocate for a post at Bourneville*] took pity on me and went to speak to you about me; I knew nothing of this. When you offered me this post, you warned me of the difficulties I would encounter, but at the time I was young, inexperienced and full of enthusiasm. I believed that my

19 Corr. CP & Minister of the Interior, DCPCAC (27 January 1913).

> love of hard work would be enough to overcome everything. I was mistaken. Now I feel ground down by my surroundings.]

It was in this letter and her article 'L'Enfance anormale', which she forwarded to the Minister, that she spoke again of her interest in improving the treatment and education of children incarcerated in the asylum.

Whatever progress Pascal made in changing the therapeutic practices of the vast Clermont Asylum, her projects of reform were halted by the advent of the Great War, which impacted disastrously on asylum life, as it did on the civilian population in general. In 1914, residents of Clermont de l'Oise witnessed the German army's triumphant sweep through the great open plains of Picardy, an advance only halted at the Marne. The inhabitants of the asylum, staff and patients, were the helpless spectators of what became a terribly drawn-out conflict. The Germans briefly occupied the town in 1914 before being driven back to the Hindenburg line slightly to the east of Compiègne, some forty kilometres away. To live in this region during the war years was to experience what the historian J. B. Duroselle characterized as: 'La catastrophe irréparable et incompréhensible' [the irreparable and incomprehensible disaster] of the German invasion.[20]

Throughout this period Pascal kept a 'War Diary', a record of her daily activities, people's reactions to the war and especially of her own frustrations with the hospital administration. In 1914, with the help of asylum staff, she helped feed the French troops in retreat. During the short German occupation of Clermont, she hid and gave medical assistance to French soldiers and helped them to cross into French territory. She was still of course in charge of her usual patients and also dealt with cases of shell-shock, a phenomenon that gave new insights to psychiatrists about the role of trauma in the onset of severe mental illness.[21]

By 1915, Pascal's relations with the Director of Clermont had deteriorated sharply, reflected in his yearly report to the Prefect that: 'Elle manque d'autorité' [She lacks authority], although he does not specify in what way.[22] In March 1915 she was promoted to the highest (exceptional) grade, with a salary of 4,500 francs, but ominous signs of administrative conflict remained: 'Il est certain que si l'avancement

20 J. B. Duroselle, *La Grande Guerre des français, l'incompréhensible catastrophe: 1914–1918* (Paris: Perrin, 1995), 27.

21 DCPCAC, 15 October 1915 and 24 March 1916.

22 DCPCAC, 9 March 1915.

était donné au mérite, Mlle Pascal ne serait pas dans les conditions pour l'obtenir, mais puisque c'est pour elle un droit, je ne vois plus aucun empêchement à ce qu'elle soit promue' [If advancement were given on merit, Mlle Pascal would certainly not gain it, but since it is hers by right, I see no impediment to her promotion].[23] These negative judgements on Pascal's professional abilities seem surprising and are contradicted at all stages of her career by medical and psychiatric colleagues. They reflect the extent to which she remained at loggerheads with the Clermont Asylum Director. This pattern would be repeated throughout her career.

Though the war figures hardly at all in Constance Pascal's Clermont official dossier, one incident recorded in it, arising from the hostilities, nearly wrecked her reputation and led her to feel increasing animosity towards the administration. On 2 July 1915, the Director wrote to inform her that he had received a complaint from a Dr Parmentier to the effect that she and Dr Demay, both members of the asylum staff, had visited private patients in Clermont, a practice explicitly forbidden by their contract of employment. Parmentier also alleged that she had made use of the hospital car for these visits and that she used her flat as a surgery for outpatients. The Director acidly reminded her that 'Il est enfin absolument contraire au règlement, que des consultations soient données à votre domicile, ce qui entraine le va et vient de personnes étrangères dans l'intérieur de l'établissement' [Lastly, it is absolutely against the rules to hold consultations at your home, which leads to the coming and going of outsiders within the establishment].[24]

Pascal's reply, 3 July 1915, was characteristically trenchant, passionate and undiplomatic:

> M. Parmentier est parti en Septembre, en abandonnant ses malades. Les Maires du pays sont venus supplier les médecins de l'asile pour soigner ces malheureux. J'ai soigné des malades à cette époque, en m'imposant une grosse fatigue. M. Parmentier, qui a agi comme un criminel, au lieu de me remercier, cherche à me faire des misères. Je ne reçois personne chez moi. Il n'y a pas de va et vient dans la maison. J'ai défendu ma porte à ces invasions. Ma clientèle ayant été gratuite, les gens en abusaient et venaient au début pour cela. J'ai des amis dans la région, des familles très connues. Les moments tragiques que nous avons connus m'ont fallu [*sic*] faire la connaissance de plusieurs

23 Corr Prefect of L'Oise & Minister of the Interior, DCPCAC (10 March 1915). 'Her right' presumably relates to length of service.

24 Corr CP & Dir DACP, 2 July 1915.

personnes. Je reçois mes amies. Je ne suis pas séquestrée à l'asile (Corr CP & Dir DACP, 3 July 1915).

> [M. Parmentier left in September, abandoning his patients. The mayors of the region came to beg us to look after these unfortunate people. I took on some of these patients, which was exhausting work. Instead of thanking me, M. Parmentier, who has acted like a criminal, is now trying to make trouble for me. I do not see patients at home. There is no coming and going in my house. I have closed my doors against such incursions. I do not charge my patients; at first, some people took advantage and came for that reason. I have friends in the locality, well-established families. As a result of the tragic times we are living in, I have become acquainted with many ladies. I receive my friends. I am not confined to the asylum.]

Two letters on Pascal's file from the grateful relatives of patients add further weight to these protestations.[25] In addition, she defended her right to receive friends in her own home. She had been obliged to ask the Director's permission to have friends to stay overnight and clearly resented her guests being vetted by the administration.

The Parmentier imbroglio took nearly a year to resolve. In March 1916, the Director, writing to the Prefect of the Department of the Oise, to whom Parmentier's complaint had also been addressed, accepted the evidence of Drs Pascal and Demay that they had only seen patients outside the asylum, on the pressing requests of the mayors of the surrounding villages, because Dr Parmentier had abandoned his post at the approach of the enemy. On this occasion, the Director was obliged to back his staff:

> Je tiens à vous assurer que les Médecins Adjoints ont toujours fait leur service avec une parfaite régularité et que je n'ai jamais constaté de négligences dans l'accomplissement de leurs fonctions. Permettez-moi enfin, Monsieur le Préfet, d'observer que M. Parmentier se borne à formuler de vagues accusations contre les Médecins-Adjoints de l'Asile sans apporter aucun fait précis d'exercice de la médecine dans la clientèle civile.[26]
>
> [I can assure you that our junior doctors have always carried out their work with perfect regularity and I have never observed any negligence in the exercise of their functions. Permit me finally, M. le Préfet, to observe that M. Parmentier limits himself to vague accusations against these junior doctors without bringing any clear evidence to justify his allegation that they practised medicine among the civilian population.]

25 DCPCAC, 15 October 1915 and 24 March 1916.

26 Corr Dir & Prefect, Département de l'Oise, Clermont DACP, 27 March 1916.

In contrast to the mundane issues raised in her administrative dossier, the journal that Constance Pascal kept throughout the war conveys the collective suffering of a population constantly under the threat of bombardment, within the almost continual sound of booming guns, as well as her own frustrations and unhappiness: 'Le cauchemar de la guerre plane au-dessus de nous toujours avec la même angoisse [...] La mort est préférable à cette vie d'attente stupide, à mon inertie surtout, car je ne fais plus rien et je suis plus malade que jamais de ne pouvoir rien faire' [The nightmare of war hangs over us all the time, bringing the same constant anguish. [...] Death would be preferable to this life of mindless waiting, to this inertia above all, for I have nothing to do and being able to do nothing is making me more ill than ever] (CP WJ, I:10). She records the loss of male staff to the army, reports of their deaths and the effects on their families. The asylum continued to function through all the chaos, although food and heating were increasingly scarce. The asylum director, who ran a tight regime, was a source of continual frustration. Pascal railed against him in the privacy of her journal, ridiculing him as a petit-bourgeois dictator.

Pascal's journal was the only outlet she possessed to express her increasing sense of oppression in her private life and the horrors of the wider military/political situation. She was profoundly conscious of the historical significance of the conflict. Many of the entries concern politics, military strategy and national attitudes, French, German and Romanian. From the perspective of the asylum, she was interested in recording patients' reactions to the bombing and the artillery fire, constantly heard in Clermont, reactions that seemed stoical because uncomprehending. Increasingly her journal became an outlet for frustrations at the hospital, where the psychiatrists' views about their patients were, she felt, largely ignored by the administration. She dwelt on her mounting unhappiness, her conviction that she was under surveillance as a single woman, and that her rooms had been searched. More generally, her patriotic feelings for France clashed with her concern for her native Romania and her fear that it would side with Germany rather than the Western Allies. Cut off from her family by the war and by her quarrels with her brother Trajan, Pascal was plunged into an abyss of homesickness and guilt. This deeply personal journal focuses on her misery and *ennui* in the suffocating atmosphere of the asylum. Yet though it served as an outlet for her most negative and frantic thoughts, a form of auto-analysis and therapeutic release, the journal is maddeningly opaque about many specific details of her life. She wrote it not as a record for posterity but to make her existence bearable.

One of Pascal's principal themes in these diaries concerns her sense of being crushed by inaction. She wanted to contribute to the war effort by driving an ambulance or even working in a munitions factory. She complained of loneliness and idleness. Yet this is deceptive. She was fully engaged in her hospital work, visited Parmentier's patients, and wrote numerous articles for scholarly journals and the popular press. Like Madeleine Pelletier, who also applied unsuccessfully to serve at the front in a medical capacity, Pascal felt that the war dramatized women's exclusion from meaningful action. 'En Angleterre les femmes vont fabriquer des munitions. Pourquoi ne pas en faire autant en France?' [In England women go to work in munitions factories. Why not do the same in France?] (CP WJ, I, 20). Meanwhile, in her day-to-day professional life, a sense of despair with the hospital bureaucracy assailed her. Excoriating the administrative 'parvenus' whose sudden access to new responsibilities had made them drunk with self-importance, she wrote scornfully with reference to the administration:

> Et ce qu'on rencontre le plus ici, ce sont les imbéciles; les imbéciles omnipotents cherchant à écraser les autres par leur autorité pathologique. [...] Et il est dur d'assister sans aucune force à ce spectacle. C'est très dur de ne rien pouvoir faire, de supporter le poids de l'autorité des imbéciles. Oh! Que c'est lourd, surtout qu'on n'a rien pour oublier ce malheur (CP WJ, I, 11–12).
>
> [All one finds here are fools, all-powerful fools who try to crush other people with their pathological authority. [...] It is very hard to stand by and watch this going on without being able to stop it. It is so hard to be able to do nothing, to have to bow to the authority of fools. How heavy a burden this is, especially when there is nothing to distract one from this misfortune.]

Every page recounted her frustration:

> Oh! Que c'est irritant et maladif cette inertie dans un asile de province où tout marche comme dans une administration dirigée par des non-valeurs. Il faut rester là en occupation passive et renoncer à tout sentiment de dignité. Cette attitude est pire que la mort. Je me sens ensevelie dans cette administration comme dans un cercueil (CP WJ, I, 14).
>
> [How infuriating and unhealthy it is to be stuck here in a provincial asylum, where all the administration is run in the name of non-values. One must carry on, passively occupied, but with no sense of

> dignity. This attitude is worse than a death sentence. Running this administration feels like being buried alive in a coffin.]

Under war conditions, the Director, who became ever more authoritarian, was the particular focus of Pascal's dislike. She observed how he had adopted military mannerisms and alleged that he spied on his employees' private lives but neglected the patients. The dormitories were dirty, mattresses and blankets filthy, there were lice in the beds and flies and mosquitoes everywhere. He refused to consult with doctors about their patients. The staff were frightened of him: 'C'est marrant de voir ce spectacle de terreur devant un petit bonhomme vulgaire, emporté, impulsif, violent' (CP WJ, I, 21–22) [It is comical to see them terrified by this vulgar, bad-tempered, impulsive, violent little man]. She rued her own weakness in allowing herself to become obsessed by the Director's pettiness, feeling that her anger should be reserved for the German enemy. To be excluded from military activity seemed terrible. She felt that her life was ebbing away, but her admiration for France increased daily:

> Et, aucune affection, pas même un peu de sympathie; pas même un peu de chaleur autour du cœur qui souffre – pas même une conversation agréable, un peu de joie pour l'esprit. Et... Vivre! Comment ai-je pu rester ici si longtemps? Comment ma destinée n'a-t-elle pas voulu que j'aie une autre vie? [...] Se passer son temps [*sic*] à soupirer, à retourner les idées, à lire entre les mots, à sentir jusqu'au profond de soi la douleur de vivre dans un milieu sans chaleur affective, sans intérêt. [...] Les Russes reculent toujours. Et rien de la Roumanie. Les Anglais ne gardent pas les tranchées perdues. Il n'y a que les Français qui sont admirables; il n'y a que les Français qui résistent et aiment mieux mourir que de se rendre (CP WJ, I, 30–32).

> [And no affection, not even a little sympathy; not even a little warmth to comfort a suffering heart — not even a pleasant conversion, a little joy for the mind. Just to *live*...! How have I managed to stay here so long? Why has fate not allowed me to live a different life? [...] One spends one's time sighing, endlessly turning over the same ideas, reading between the lines, feeling to the depths of one's soul how painful it is to live in a place without warmth or affection, without any interest. [...] The Russians are in retreat. Not a word from Romania. The English abandon their trenches. Only the French resist – they are admirable: they would sooner die than surrender.]

Meanwhile civilians complained about war conditions and the behaviour of French soldiers in the recaptured zones. Reports emerged of furniture being looted for firewood from houses near the front line. Pascal's sympathies were emphatically with the soldiers:

> On demande que les soldats fassent des sacrifices pour nous défendre; verser leur sang pour garder la France à nous et on leur reproche de se chauffer avec les pieds des fauteuils. [...] On leur doit tout! Sans eux, les mêmes choses appartiendraient aux Boches (CP, WJ I, 36).
>
> [We expect soldiers to make sacrifices to defend us, to shed their blood to keep France for the French, and then we reproach them for warming themselves with chair legs. [...] We owe them everything! Without them all these objects would be in the hands of the Hun.]

And still the overwhelming feeling of inertia and boredom in the (exceptionally, dated) entry of 9 June 1915:

> J'étouffe ici. Je dois m'en aller. Je voudrais habiter Paris, ce foyer de solidarité, ce nid de générosité. Cette vision d'égoïsme, d'avarice m'écrase. J'ai continuellement un serrement du cœur, une crispation générale physique et morale. Ça me diminue, ça m'affaiblit (CP WJ, I, 46).
>
> [This place is stifling me. I must get out. I want to live in Paris, that centre of solidarity, that hearth of generosity. The sight of all the egoism and avarice here are destroying me. I feel constant heart pangs and a tension that is both physical and moral, which diminishes and enfeebles me.]

In stark contrast to this sense of 'total lifelessness', a local newspaper article dated 14 March 1915 praises Pascal's activity and courage in succouring the wounded:

> A six heures vive fusillade dans la direction du bois. Les Français quoique moins nombreux défendent le terrain pied à pied. Deux sont tués, trois autres blessés. Ces trois derniers réussissent à gagner Fitz-James. Le premier est transporté à l'hospice par les soins de M. Mazille, conseiller municipal de Clermont, charcutier au Pont de Pierre. Le second vient échouer sur les marches de l'église de Fitz-James. Il est secouru par Mme Lejuste et transporté au presbytère avec l'aide de Mlles Bellegou et Godard. Mlle la doctoresse Pascal qui durant cette période fit preuve d'un grand dévouement à l'égard des malades civiles et militaires, lui prodigua les soins les plus empressés. [...] Au cours de ses visites Mlle Pascal avait rencontré des Allemands qui lui avaient dit: 'Françouses, trente-six capout [sic] au bois St-Jean.' Mlle Pascal n'hésite pas une seule minute. Avec une voiture accompagnée de MM. Lefebvre, Norbert et Mercier, elle part dans les lignes allemandes à la recherche des morts et des blessés. Heureusement, les Boches avaient comme toujours beaucoup exagéré. Il y avait en tout deux morts qui furent inhumés dans le cimetière du

village avec l'argent de deux généreuses personnes.[27] [*Written in pencil in the margin: 'Mlle Pascal'.*]

[At six o'clock, there was a loud fusillade in the direction of the woods. Although much fewer in number, the French defended the terrain inch by inch. Two were killed, three wounded. These three managed to reach Fitz-James. The first was taken to the hospital by M. Mazille, a butcher from Pont de Pierre who is on the town council of Clermont. The second collapsed on the steps of the Fitz-James church. Mme Lejuste came to his aid and he was carried into the presbytery with the help of Mlles Bellegou and Godard. Mlle la *doctoresse* Pascal, who showed great devotion to both civilian and military patients throughout this period, cared for him most assiduously. [...] During her rounds, Mlle Pascal had met some Germans who had told her: 'Thirty-six Frenches *kaput* in St Jean woods'. Without a moment's hesitation, Mlle Pascal took a car and, together with MM. Lefebvre Norbert and Mercier, set off towards the German lines to find the dead and wounded. Fortunately the Huns had exaggerated, as usual. In all there were just two dead, and they were interred in the village cemetery with money donated by two generous persons.] [*Written in pencil in the margin: 'Mlle Pascal'.*]

At last, in the summer of 1915, Pascal's journal records a complete shift in tone, with this telling comment: 'Aujourd'hui j'ai causé avec un homme intelligent mais qui a, comme tous les hommes intelligents, des partis pris' [I had a talk today with an intelligent man – though, like all intelligent men, he has his prejudices] (CP WJ, I, 46). Thanks to the proximity of Clermont to the front line, part of the French General Staff was quartered at Clermont de l'Oise in the Fitz-James Château, adjacent to the section of the hospital where Pascal worked. As she had noted to the asylum director in the same summer: 'The tragic times that we have witnessed have allowed me to make the acquaintance of several people.' The 'intelligent man' noted above, who in her journal stands in marked contrast to her exasperated remarks about the asylum Director, was General Justin Mengin, Commander of the 6th Army Brigade.

The conversations with General Mengin that Pascal records in her journal reveal a sudden transformation in her mood. She had found someone with whom she could discuss the war intelligently and debate wider issues. She had also discovered the love of her life. But though she records lively debates between herself and Mengin on war and politics, she reveals not a glimmer of what must have been a growing mutual romantic and sexual attraction:

27 *Gazette de L'Oise*, DCPCAC (14 March 1915).

Il m'a dit qu'il est étonné de voir qu'à ces moments difficiles il n'y a pas un homme, pas un qui ait l'étincelle divine ni en stratégie ni en politique. – Et Joffre? – Un commis. – Comment? Et la victoire de la Marne? Oh! Oui c'est beau, oui, j'ai du respect pour lui mais il n'a fait que réaliser une vielle idée de l'École Polytechnique. – Eh bien. L'avoir appliquée à mesure de son âme, n'est-ce pas l'étincelle géniale? De tous les actes instinctifs, créateurs, généreux n'y a-t-il pas toujours des prémisses connues? L'étincelle ne réside-t-elle pas de l'idée exacte dans l'application qui réalise les tendances des prémisses? Joffre a appliqué génialement l'idée ancienne d'affermir sur la Marne; un autre aurait eu cette idée mais il n'aurait pas su trouver le moment, les circonstances. Et puis n'avoir pas douté de la France, n'est-ce pas encore une force de génie? Il a gardé sa lucidité dans le désarroi des politiciens. N'est-ce pas là une force de génie? Mon grand homme intéressant m'a dit qu'il n'y avait pas d'hommes politiques capables en France en ce moment; ce sont de bons commis' (CP WJ, I, 47).

[He told me he is amazed to see that in these difficult times there is not one man in either military strategy or politics who has a spark of inspiration. – 'How about Joffre?' – 'A pen-pusher.' – 'Really? What about the Battle of the Marne?' – 'Well, yes, that was good, I have lots of respect for him, but all he was doing is carrying out an old idea from the École Polytechnique [*the military college*]'. – 'Yes but knowing when and how to apply an old idea – surely that is the sign of genius? Isn't every instinctive, creative, inspired act based on a known premise? The spark of genius consists in applying it in exactly the right way to bring out its potential. Joffre took the old idea of consolidation on the Marne; anyone else could have had the same idea; he knew how to seize the moment, find exactly the right circumstances. – And he never stopped believing in France; that's another sign of his genius, isn't it? And he kept a clear head when the politicians were giving up; surely that's another.' But my interesting great man told me that there are no politicians worth their salt in France just now; nothing but competent pen-pushers.]

This dialogue continues for several pages ranging over military strategy, politics and popular responses to the war. Pascal had encountered an intellectual equal, with whom she did not necessarily agree – indeed she makes a point of showing her dissent from his opinions – but with whom it was possible to talk intelligently. She had long been starved of the kind of intellectual companionship she had known in Paris. The account of her 'interesting man' is sardonic, yet she is evidently very taken with him. He shares, Pascal thinks, the characteristic scepticism of the French. 'Cet esprit critique négative est bien français, cet esprit qui explique tout, analyse tout ce qui est mauvais et laisse à coté ce qui est bon' [This negative critical attitude is very French: it explains everything, analyses everything wrong and leaves aside everything good] (CP WJ, I, 47). Her lengthy account of these conversations and her meditations on them traces a dialectical movement that both conceals and reveals the progress of an unlikely love affair. Life had begun again at last.

Justin Mengin, ebullient, charming and intelligent, was the son of a schoolteacher at Colmy, a village in the Department of Meurthe and Moselle, and a typical product of the meritocratic culture encouraged under the Third Republic. As a boy he showed early intellectual promise, attending the College at Thionville before winning a place, first at the Lycée Charlemagne in Paris and then a scholarship at the prestigious École Polytechnique in Paris, graduating in 1876. His school certificate gives the following statistics of his appearance: height 1.76 meters, brown hair, blue eyes, oval face. He was ranked 98th out of 252 students in his class and on entry to the Artillery School, 35th out of 137. He was considered a good student.

When he made the acquaintance of Mlle la *doctoresse* Pascal, General Mengin was fifty-nine years old and she was thirty-eight. Photographs taken in the war years show a robust man with the Clemenceau moustaches of the day, astride a horse, looking every inch the general. He had a successful career behind him, having risen steadily through the ranks. He was made lieutenant in 1878, captain in 1884, squadron leader in 1898, lieutenant colonel in 1904, colonel in 1907, then a two-year posting in Algeria (beginning February 1912) followed by promotion to general of brigade in May 1912 and general of division in 1914. He served in the artillery and was attached to the General Staff. In 1902 he had received special commendation in a 'lettre d'éloges' [letter of commendation] from the minister of war, General André, for the zeal and competence with which he had managed the technical section to which he was assigned. Mengin was admired by his superior officers who, in their reports, commented on his competence, intelligence and zeal. 'C'est un collaborateur hors ligne, d'une activité toujours en excitation, outre d'un caractère charmant et d'une bonne volonté à toute épreuve' [He is an outstanding colleague, full of energy, always active, with a charming personality and endlessly obliging to his friends].[28] He was warmly commended for his management of the engineering workshop and as being calm, thoughtful, methodical and open to new ideas – in short, an officer of the first rank.

General Mengin was also a married man. It is possible that he first met Constance Pascal when he came to consult her about his wife,

28 Dossier Justin Mengin, AHMD.

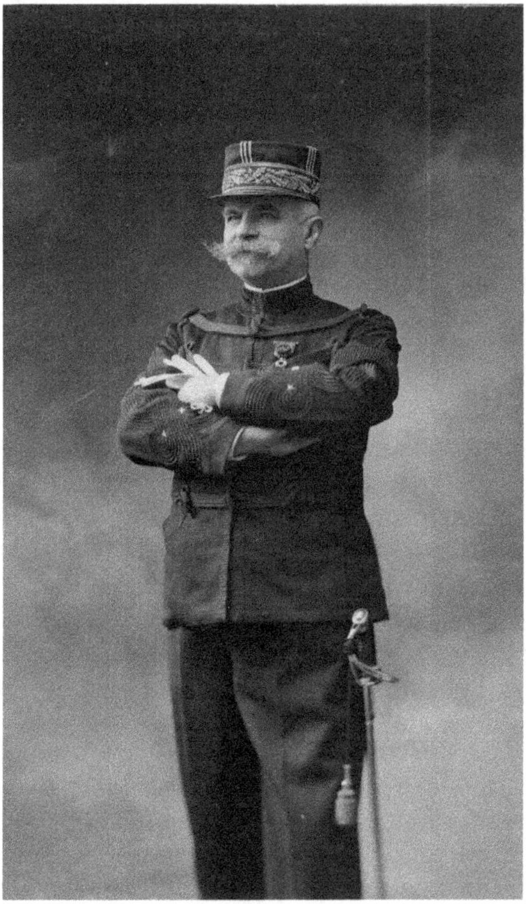

Fig 2. General Justin Mengin

Marie Gabrielle Nicolas Mengin who, four years later in 1920, would be interned in the asylum of Evreux in Normandy and who may already then have been suffering from mental illness.[29] Alternatively they may have been introduced through mutual friends in Paris, the Bouvard sisters. Was marriage ever a possibility? Under French law Mengin could not divorce if his wife was detained in a mental hospital.[30] We know she was a patient at Evreux Asylum in 1920,

29 Information supplied by the Bureau de la Gestion des Malades, Centre Hospitalier Spécialisé de Navarre, Évreux, 22 May 2003.

30 See Laure Murat, *La Maison du Docteur Blanche* (Paris: Hachette, 2001), 290–92. The law of 1884, which liberalized divorce in France, forbade it in the case of patients interned in asylums, a measure intended to protect the interests of the mentally ill.

but she may have been interned in another hospital previously. As for Pascal, had she married, she would have been relegated to the status of a minor, incompatible with directing a psychiatric ward. She would have been disqualified from exercising the civil and legal responsibilities of an asylum doctor.[31]

Marie Gabrielle Nicolas was forty-six when she married Justin Mengin in 1906; he was fifty-one. They had cohabited for twenty years prior to their marriage. Mlle Nicolas had held a responsible position in the Crédit Lyonnais bank, from 1889 to 1905, as head of the women's services. The officer who vetted her suitability as an army wife spoke of her good character: 'Ces renseignements recueillis sur la conduite et la moralité de la future épouse sont excellents – très bien élevée, menant avec le Colonel une existence parfaitement régulière et correcte, Mlle Nicolas jouit de l'estime de tout son entourage qui, d'ailleurs, la croit mariée' [The information gathered on the conduct and morality of the future wife is excellent – very well brought up, leading a perfectly correct and respectable life with the Colonel, Mlle Nicolas enjoys the esteem of all who know her and who in fact believe her to be married already]. [32]

What disasters subsequently overtook Marie Nicolas Mengin are not known. If we believe the army's vetting officer, she and the Colonel had enjoyed a long and stable relationship. Yet by 1916, ten years after her marriage, she suffered a severe breakdown and her husband had fathered a child by France's first woman psychiatrist. Given the outward respectability demanded by both lovers' professional positions, Justin Mengin and Constance Pascal organized a complex structure of subterfuge to hide the nature of their relationship and the subsequent birth of their child, a deception that lasted until their deaths. It is impossible to say whether Marie Gabrielle fell ill before, during or after the General's affair with Constance Pascal. We have no independent testimony as to her illness save in his will, where he mentions the expenses attached to maintaining her at the Evreux asylum and the dates of her internment.[33]

31 In the Avant-propos', *Chagrins d'amour et psychoses*, iv, Chazaud notes that Pascal's 'statut de femme interdisait le mariage sous peine d'être disqualifiée par la "minorisation" de l'épouse pour exercer, en ce temps-là, les fonctions expertales et plus généralement, de responsabilités civiles et légales.' [Pascal's status as a woman prohibited marriage for fear of disqualification, due to the status of wives as minors, from her professional functions and more generally from her civil and legal responsibilities.] See also: Édouard Toulouse, 'La femme et les fonctions publiques' DMP, BMD (n. d.).

32 Rapport du Capitaine Blaye, Paris, DJM (3 September 1906).

33 Justin Mengin, 'Ceci est mon Testament', PRFP.

If General Mengin owed his meeting with Constance Pascal to a consultation over his wife's psychiatric illness, he may have been referred to her because she was an acknowledged expert in early dementia and had published an article in 1906, 'Délire des préjudices préséniles', on mental disturbances in menopausal women, summing up the work of Kraepelin.[34] Marie Gabrielle may have experienced the acute anxiety suffered by some menopausal patients, a state deemed irreversible but which, according to Pascal's article, did not count as complete insanity:

> Les perturbations du retour d'âge ont été décrites par de nombreux auteurs. [...] Peu à peu émergent les idées de préjudice qui peuvent être réparties en trois groupes distincts, suivant que le malade s'imagine éprouver du dommage soit dans sa santé, soit dans sa propriété, soit dans son affection conjugale.
>
> A. *Idées de préjudice portant sur la santé ou idées hypochondriaques.* Ce sont celles qui s'installent les premières. Les malades se plaignent des troubles nerveux les plus divers: sanglots, tressaillements convulsifs, vertiges, douleurs erratiques, rêves agités, faiblesse, enflure, craquements dans la tête, etc. [...]
>
> B. *Idées de préjudice portant sur la propriété ou idées de persécution.* Leur apparition est ultérieure à celles des précédentes. On change les vêtements, les objets, le piano du malade; on le vole; on éraille ses miroirs, ses meubles, les plats de la cuisine; on lui apporte de la poussière dans ses appartements; il y a des voleurs dans la maison; [...] les médecins préparent des mixtures mystérieuses pour provoquer artificiellement en lui une maladie qu'ils étudieront.
>
> C. *Idées de préjudice portant sur l'affection conjugale ou délire d'infidélité conjugale.* Le nombre de ces idées les place parfois au premier plan du tableau symptomatique. Le mari fréquente toutes les femmes qu'il peut; il fait l'œil par derrière son journal à sa voisine, échange des regards entendus avec les jeunes filles qu'il rencontre, se commande une femme pour chacun de ses voyages, est en correspondance avec les amies de sa fille; les morceaux de billets trouvés dans la caisse à papier sont autant de pièces à conviction. [...]
>
> Quant à l'avenir de ces malades, l'auteur insiste sur ce point que tout en étant progressif, leur affaiblissement intellectuel n'arrive pas à la démence complète. Jamais non plus il ne survient ni guérison ni même une amélioration durable (Pascal, 'Délire', 573–75).

34 Emil Kraepelin, *Psychiatrie*, 8e édition (Leipzig: J.A. Barth, 1906); Constance Pascal, 'Délire des préjudices préséniles', *L'Encéphale*, I: 6 (25 November 1906), 571–72.

> [Disturbances of the change of life have been described by numerous authors. [...] Bit by bit obsessive ideas of harm emerge; these can be divided into three distinct groups: the patient imagines experiencing harm either to her health, to her property, or to her conjugal affections.
>
> A. *Ideas of harm bearing on health, or hypochondriacal ideas.* These are the first to become established. Patients complain of the most diverse nervous troubles: sobs, convulsive trembling, dizziness, aches and pains, disturbed dreams, weakness, swelling, creaking noises in the head, etc. [...]
>
> B. *Ideas of harm bearing on property, or ideas of persecution.* These come after the ideas just described. Someone has moved the patient's clothes, objects or piano; she is being robbed; her mirrors, furniture or dishes have been scratched; dust has been brought into the apartment; there are thieves in the house; [...] doctors are preparing mysterious potions that will make her ill, so that they can study the effects.
>
> C. *Ideas of harm bearing on marital affection or the delusion of marital infidelity.* These ideas are so numerous that often they are at the forefront of the symptomatic picture. Her husband is consorting with all the women he can find, making eyes behind his newspaper at the woman next to him or exchanging meaningful glances with any girl he meets; each time he travels he takes a different woman with him; he is corresponding with his daughter's best friends; torn-up tickets in the waste paper basket are so many pieces of evidence against him. [...]
>
> As for the future of these patients, the author insists that while it may be a progressive condition, *their gradual loss of intellectual coherence does not amount to complete insanity. On the other hand, there is no question of a cure or even an improvement.*][35]

If these were the fears experienced by Marie Gabrielle, they would, ironically, prove self-fulfilling. Her husband, though far from the lecherous figure imagined by Kraepelin's patients, if his official dossier is any guide, did enact a drama of 'marital infidelity'. However applicable the above diagnosis might have been, the amorous triangle emerging from this web of relationships also has a clear social context. There is, first, the fact of the late marriage of Marie Gabrielle Nicolas and Justin Mengin in 1906. This certainly did not reflect the model of family values promulgated in Third Republic France, yet neither Marie Nicolas nor Justin Mengin appear to have been social rebels, indeed their background and general behaviour were solidly petit-bourgeois. Their late marriage was not the idiosyncratic choice of the

35 I have used the feminine gender in the English translation where appropriate as the context refers to female patients.

two contracting partners, but a situation typical of officers and their partners in the French Army, where so many restrictions were placed on the possibility of marriage that in the mid nineteenth century 34% of officers were unmarried at the age of 50, compared with about 12% of men in the civilian population.[36] Many officers, unable to marry, simply cohabited, as seems to have been the case with Justin Mengin and Marie Nicolas.

Since the late seventeenth century a strong prejudice had existed in the high command against officers marrying. Marriage was seen as likely to ensnare them in extra expense and as making them far less likely to wish to risk their lives in battle. This general prejudice contributed to the raft of legislation and military rules governing officers' private lives throughout the nineteenth and into the early twentieth centuries. All military personnel were deprived by law of the right freely to contract marriage. This was an important exception to the French revolution's abolition of feudal impediments to marriage. As one writer puts it: 'Le mariage des militaires est soumis à des conditions restrictives nécessitées par les exigences de la vie militaire, le souci du maintien de la discipline et de la dignité du corps d'officiers et de sous-officiers' [The marriage of military personnel is subject to restrictive conditions made necessary by the exigencies of military life and the need to safeguard discipline and the dignity of the corps of officers and junior officers].[37] An imperial decree of 16 June 1808 had stipulated that no officer could marry without obtaining permission in writing from the Minister of War. If an officer married without permission, he would be stripped of his salary and pension rights for himself and his family.

Applying this strict ruling proved complex. What were the grounds for refusing a request for marriage? The most contentious proved to be the requirement, first instituted in 1817, that the intended bride must possess a dowry commensurate with the rank of the husband-to-be. By 1843, the sum required was at least 1,200 francs of private income per year, not in the form of a life annuity. The rationale for this rule rested on the fear that married officers would contract unmanageable debts, or that their widows and children would be a charge on the army. The other major stipulation was that the wife must not be employed. This ruling reflected snobbery against officers marrying into a 'trade' and ignored the growing number of women

36 See William Serman, *Officiers français dans la nation 1814–1914* (Paris: Aubier Montaigne, 1982), pp. 145–183 and Claude Croubois, *L'Officier français des origines à nos jours* (Saint-Jean-d'Angely: Éditions Bordessoules, 1987), 232–34.

37 Oscar Berger-Leuvrault, *Dictionnaire militaire* (Paris: Alcan, 1910), 1844.

in professional posts, who were excluded as wives unless they gave up their careers. An article in *La Fronde*, written from a strongly anti-clerical perspective, argued that such rules demonstrated that the army wanted officers to marry only docile and socially conservative women:

> Le prétexte sous lequel on a conservé dans l'armée de la République l'ancien système du recrutement des femmes des militaires, est de protéger les officiers contre les entraînements de la passion. [...] Mais la vérité est que le recrutement des femmes d'officiers n'a d'autre but que de préserver la caste militaire de toute contamination d'esprit civil démocratique. [...] Les champs de bataille où l'on gagne des galons et des croix, sont les salons des femmes d'officiers. Il importe donc que la direction de ces lieux de gloire ne soit confiée qu'à des personnes sûres, et élevées dans les bons principes. Il importe par-dessus tout qu'elles aillent régulièrement à confesse, et que la Congrégation soit en dernier ressort la seule maîtresse de l'avancement et la vraie dispensatrice des grades et des commandements. Du moins ces dispositions importent à la gloire de Dieu et au bénéfice de son représentant à Rome.[38]

> [The excuse given by the Army of the Republic for retaining the old system of recruiting army wives is that it saves officers from the snares of passion. [...] But the truth is that the recruitment of officers' wives has no other aim than to preserve the military class from being contaminated by the democratic spirit of the civilian world. [...] Officers' wives' salons are the battlefields in which stripes and medals are earned. It is essential, therefore, that the management of these fields of glory should be confined to reliable persons, brought up with the right principles. It is especially essential that these women go to confession regularly and that the Church be the supreme arbiter of promotions and the true distributor of ranks and commissions. At least these arrangements are essential for the glory of God and the fortune of his representative in Rome.]

It was not until 1900 that General André, Minister of War, a strong republican and impatient of the social distinctions encouraged by the army ethos, dispensed with the dowry requirement, though not the vetting of prospective wives or the requirement to seek permission to marry.[39] Even after André's reform, permission for marriage depended on the subjective opinions of senior officers. Did

38 Bradamante, 'Le Mariage des officiers', *La Fronde* (28 December 1901). Bradamante was a warrior heroine from Ariosto's *Orlando furioso*.

39 *Bulletin officiel* (2e semester, 1900), 1577–1578. For a critical view of General André's tenure as Minister of War see Alistair Horne, *The French Army and Politics 1870–1970* (London: Macmillan, 1984), 25–30.

they, as many did, disapprove of cohabiting couples (*concubinage*), or did they take a more relaxed and pragmatic view? Justin Mengin and Marie Nicolas lived out a domestic situation imposed by these military regulations. Mengin did not apply to marry until 1906, two years after he was made Lieutenant Colonel with a salary of 7,200 francs. Having no private income, it was not till then that he was able to afford a wife. His salary rose to 9,000 francs in 1907, when he was promoted to Colonel, to 12,600 when he became Brigadier General and to 18,900 francs when he became General of Division in 1914.

Marie Nicolas gave up her post at the Crédit Lyonnais in 1905, no doubt to qualify for marriage to an officer. She had saved a small dowry, but was released from the need for a larger one by General André's reform. Captain Blaye, who vetted her, was evidently sympathetic to the couple, stressing their respectability and the fact that Marie Nicolas was suitable officer-wife material. She had had no children during her twenty-year relationship with Justin Mengin. Was she ever to discover that another woman had a child by her husband? Could this have been a precipitating cause of her breakdown, or had mental illness overtaken her before Mengin met Constance Pascal? These questions can probably never be answered unless hospital records are made available, but the couple practised such perfect discretion that it seems unlikely that Marie Mengin knew of the affair. Even Justin Mengin's remaining family in Colmy, a sister, and her two sons, knew nothing of Mlle Pascal or of her daughter Jeanne, though Mengin frequently visited his Lorraine relatives and remained warmly attached to his child to the end of his life.

It is evident from Pascal's letters to her sister-in-law Marie that she had thought a great deal about maternity and the upbringing of children and that she longed for a child. Following a visit to her aunt 'Mite' she analysed the latter's maternal preoccupations with words that may well have reflected her own deeper anxieties:

> Ses sentiments maternels un peu trop tardifs l'éloignent de ses parents. [...] J'ai pitié de ce pauvre cœur de femme qui n'a jamais été mère et qui a été toute sa vie assoiffée de maternité. [...] Elle ne se rend pas compte du sentiment maternel presque morbide par son excès et par l'oubli des autres. [...] C'est bien triste une vie vide (Corr CP & MP, PRFP, 8 September 1912).

> [Her maternal feelings, which arose somewhat too late in life, are estranging her from her family. [...] I pity this poor woman, who has never had a child yet has thirsted for motherhood all her life. [...] She is not aware how extreme, even morbid her maternal feelings are,

both in their excess and in the neglect of others that they cause in her. [...] how sad it is to have an empty life.]

Pascal realized she was pregnant sometime in November 1915 (she probably conceived in October). She was both terrified and elated, writing in her journal: 'Si tard mais tant désiré' [So late, but so much desired]. Her decision to bear a child was courageous and possibly foolhardy. It could have had catastrophic consequences for her career and her reputation, but her thirst for motherhood, as she said of her aunt, over-rode considerations of prudence. She had experienced enough of 'an empty life'. She did not seem to have contemplated an abortion which, given her medical contacts, she easily could have arranged, even though the laws against abortion in France were strict, Article 317 of the Penal Code making abortion illegal and punishable by a custodial sentence.[40] Without a doubt her situation was daunting. Here she was, in 1916, in mid-war, a single woman due to give birth to a baby whose father was a married senior officer. Secrecy was absolutely necessary, as of course was the need to hide her pregnancy.

In March 1916, with the baby due in July, she applied for, and was granted, a month's leave, as of 1 April, for 'raisons de santé' [on health grounds]. The director explained this leave retrospectively in her administrative dossier as 'une opération chirurgicale qui l'a tenue éloignée de son service pendant plus de trois mois et qui l'oblige encore à des précautions' [an operation that has kept her away from work for more than three months and which still requires her to take precautions].[41] By April, however, it was clearly imperative that she leave Clermont before her pregnancy became visible. She declined to take leave of the Director in person (as would have been customary) on the grounds of her 'ill health', but more probably to hide her changing appearance. A protracted and acrimonious dispute with him about the amount of wood she burned in her apartment from February to March reveals her sense of vulnerability. She first denied that there was any excess consumption, whilst complaining bitterly of the cold, and then, recognizing that the Director held receipts to prove how much wood she had used, she wrote a letter of apology mixed with further complaints. One day later, in a repentant mood, but also ironically obsequious, she referred obliquely, though the Director could not have known this, to her child's approaching birth:

40 Gordon, *IF*, 134–36.

41 Corr Prefect of the Oise & Dir, Clermont DACP (30 March 1916); (October 1916).

> Il est temps que je quitte la maison. Je perturbe le bon ordre du budget; je suis impardonnable. Permettez-moi de vous proposer de payer ce que j'ai pris en trop. [...] Je pars ces jours-ci vers un inconnu qui ne m'épouvante pas mais qui m'attriste beaucoup. J'aurais désirée aller vous voir et vous dire adieu. Fatiguée, devenue impressionnable comme une petite fille, je ne peux affronter l'indignation du bon administrateur. Permettez-moi de vous faire mes adieux par lettre (Corr CP & Dir, Clermont, DACP, April 1916).

> [It is high time I left this institution. I am causing problems in the management of your budget. This is unforgivable of me. Allow me to pay for the extra wood I have used. [...] I will depart any day now towards an unknown destiny, which does not frighten me but does make me very sad. I should have liked to say goodbye to you; but I am exhausted and, feeling as sensitive as a little girl, I cannot face the irritation of the worthy administrator. Permit me therefore to take my leave by this letter.]

What is revealing about the wood-burning saga is the emotional tenor of her letters suggesting the pressure she was under. The strain of concealing her pregnancy, and the 'unknown' to which she refers, bearing an illegitimate child at the age of thirty-nine (all of which was also 'unknown' to the Director), must have been almost overwhelming.

With the assistance of Jeanne Streicher and General Mengin, Pascal booked into a Paris clinic. On 22 April, writing from the Maison de Santé, 219 rue Vercengétorix, Paris XIVe, with her leave nearly expired but the baby not due until July, Pascal applied for a further three months' absence, sending medical certificates as justification.[42] She evidently had a sympathetic doctor prepared to testify vaguely to gynaecological problems. Leave was granted. She finally returned to her post at Clermont on 16 August, one month after the birth of her daughter. Jeanne Pascal was born on 17 July 1916. On the birth certificate is recorded: 'Père et mère non dénommés' [Parents unknown].[43] Initially Pascal sent the baby to a 'pépinière' [nursery] but within a few months she took over her care and formally fostered her. Though brought up by her natural mother and maintaining an affectionate relationship with her father, whom she knew as her godfather, Jeanne Pascal was never legally recognized by either parent.

42 Maison de Santé, 219 rue Vercingétorix, Paris XIVe, Clermont DACP.

43 Bulletin de Naissance, Ville de Paris XIVème Arrondissement, Jeanne Madeleine Marie, PRFP (17 July 1916).

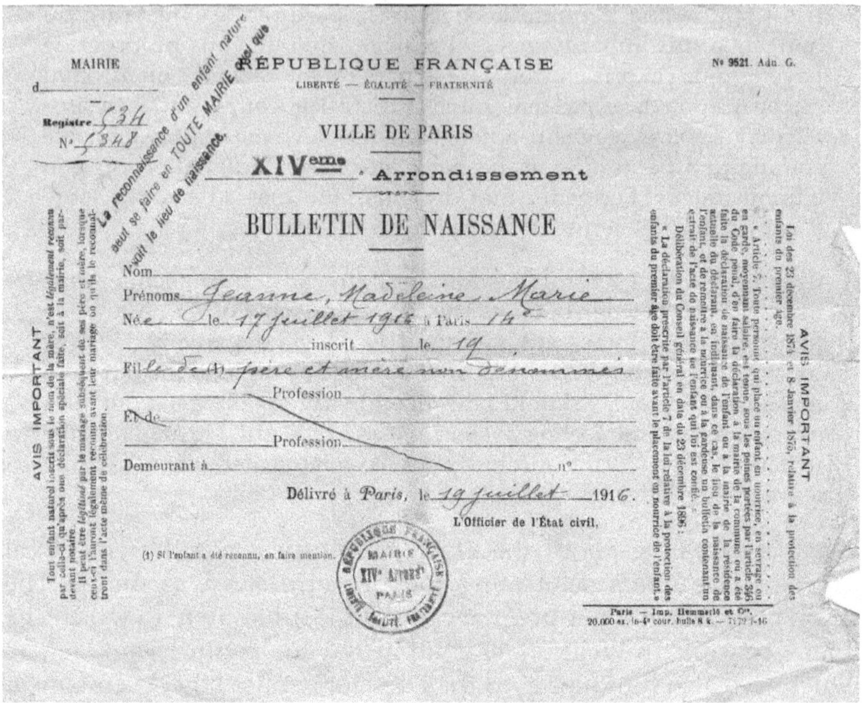

MAIRIE

d

Registre 534

N° 5348

RÉPUBLIQUE FRANÇAISE

LIBERTÉ — ÉGALITÉ — FRATERNITÉ

N° 9521. Adm. G.

La reconnaissance d'un enfant naturel peut se faire en TOUTE MAIRIE quel que soit le lieu de naissance.

VILLE DE PARIS

XIVème Arrondissement

BULLETIN DE NAISSANCE

Nom

Prénoms Jeanne, Madeleine, Marie

Née le 17 juillet 1916 à Paris 14e

inscrit le 19

Fille de (1) père et mère non dénommés

Profession

Et de

Profession

Demeurant à n°

Délivré à Paris, le 19 juillet 1916.

L'Officier de l'État civil.

(1) Si l'enfant a été reconnu, en faire mention.

MAIRIE XIVe Arrondt PARIS — RÉPUBLIQUE FRANÇAISE — LIBERTÉ ÉGALITÉ FRATERNITÉ

AVIS IMPORTANT

Tout enfant naturel inscrit sous le nom de la mère, n'est *légalement reconnu* par celle-ci qu'après une déclaration spéciale faite, soit à la mairie, soit par-devant notaire.

Il peut être *légitimé* par le mariage subséquent de ses père et mère, lorsque ceux-ci l'auront légalement reconnu avant leur mariage ou qu'ils le reconnaîtront dans l'acte même de célébration.

AVIS IMPORTANT

Loi des 23 décembre 1874 et 8 Janvier 1875, relative à la protection des enfants du premier âge.

« Article 7. Toute personne qui place un enfant en nourrice, en sevrage ou en garde, moyennant salaire, est tenue, sous les peines portées par l'article 346 du Code pénal, d'en faire la déclaration à la mairie de la commune où a été faite la déclaration de naissance de l'enfant ou à la mairie de la résidence actuelle du déclarant, en indiquant, dans ce cas, le lieu de la naissance de l'enfant, et de remettre à la nourrice ou à la gardeuse un bulletin contenant un extrait de l'acte de naissance de l'enfant qui lui est confié. »

Délibération du Conseil général en date du 23 décembre 1886 :

« La déclaration prescrite par l'article 7 de la loi relative à la protection des enfants du premier âge doit être faite avant le placement en nourrice de l'enfant. »

Paris — Imp. Hemmerlé et Cie.
20,000 ex. in-4° cour. bulle 8 k. — 7172 1-16

Fig 3. Jeanne Pascal's birth certificate: 'father and mother unknown'.

Pascal was not alone during this crisis. Her good friend Jeanne Streicher supported her, in spite of her own rigid moral code, which must have been greatly stretched to accommodate her admired friend. She strongly disapproved of Pascal's entanglement with the General, but was loyal to her and her daughter throughout her life. She became the baby's guardian, as did both the parents at the moment of adoption some seven years later. And what of the General? From his administrative dossier we know that he too took sick leave from April until July, suffering from a wound to his foot. General Foch granted the leave personally and may have known of reasons other than a war wound to account for it.

Pascal and Mengin's overriding preoccupation with regard to their love affair and its consequences, the birth of Jeanne in 1916, was to maintain absolute secrecy. Whether or not the Director of Clermont had any suspicions to account for Pascal's illness at the time and her need to take extended leave, nothing emerges from her personal dossier at Clermont to suggest it. What is perhaps even more remarkable is that Pascal succeeded in hiding the facts of Jeanne's parentage from public knowledge throughout her lifetime, a story only revealed in 2001.[44] To appreciate fully the anxieties under which Pascal and Mengin both laboured, one must revisit both French law under the Napoleonic Code and the moral climate of the period, insofar as it bore on the professional classes. Adultery and illegitimacy were not unknown at the turn of the century; twenty-four out of one hundred children were born out of wedlock. As far as middle-class morality was concerned, bourgeois France at the beginning of the century was not puritanical: but it tended to be prudish.[45] Social denial and ostracism, particularly towards the 'guilty' woman were the norm. As Nelly Roussel, the feminist and birth control advocate, wrote in 1904 attacking the French Civil Code as it applied to unwed mothers:

> Tu seras seule à supporter le poids de ce que les hypocrisies bourgeoises appelleront avec mépris ta 'faute'. Et ce ne sera pas assez pour l'expier, des tortures physiques que constituent pour toi, femme, une sorte de rançon de l'amour [...] Non ! la Société gardienne de la 'morale' viendra ajouter tous ses raffinements ! Elle te réserve, pour te mieux châtier, l'abandon, le mépris, la misère ; l'impossibilité de te refaire, par le travail, une vie heureuse et libre.[46]
>
> [You will bear the brunt alone of what bourgeois hypocrisy will contemptuously call your 'fall'. And you will not succeed in expiating it through the ordinary physical torments that you, as a woman, bear as the price of love. [...] No: society, the guardian of 'morality', will add its own refinements. It reserves for you the public punishment of abandonment, contempt and destitution, and makes it impossible for you to recover a happy and free life through work.]

It was true that Mengin had committed adultery, compounded by the fact that Mengin's wife was an asylum patient. However, adultery by a married man was only a crime if committed in the matrimonial home; for a wife, on the other hand, it was a crime punishable by prison, in any location.[47] From a legal point of view,

44 Rees, 'ÀPCP', 184.

45 Françoise Giroud, *Une Femme honorable* (Paris: Fayard, 1981), 219.

46 Nelly Roussel (1904), speech protesting against the Civil Code, on the anniversary of its centennial celebration, 'Protestation Féministe contre la Célébration du Centenaire du Code Civil', La Fronde, no. 2106 (1 November 1904), quoted in Susan Groag Bell and Karen M. Offen, *Women, the Family, and Freedom: the Debate in Documents*, vol. II, 1880–1950 (Stanford California: Stanford University Press, 1983), 135. I wish particularly to thank Karen Offen for making the French text available to me.

47 See Roderick Phillips, *Putting Asunder: a History of Divorce in Western Society* (Cambridge: Cambridge University Press, 1988), 422–28.

Mengin and Pascal were not in danger of criminal sanctions but rather of social opprobrium. Their child, who would be classed as an 'enfant adultérin' [child of adultery] if her origins were known, would not have rights of parental inheritance and would be the object of social stigma.[48] Given that Mengin was a senior officer in the military and Pascal was the first woman to hold the professional position of a psychiatrist in France, the publicity that followed, were their affair made public, would have fatally compromised Pascal. In the public mind errant husbands were less tainted than the women with whom they consorted. In an extra-marital relationship, only the woman risked her reputation.[49] When one recalls that as a young woman Pascal had enjoyed favourable publicity in the press as a female 'first' in psychiatry, praised not only for her beauty and brains but her decorous, respectable demeanour, public knowledge of her affair and the illegitimate child resulting from it would have cost her not only her reputation but also her career.

Particular difficulties attached themselves to women taking up a role in the professions. The idea of women in public remained deeply associated with the idea of prostitution, 'les femmes publiques', the 'oldest profession'. Proudhon had famously offered women a choice: to be 'ménagères ou courtisanes' [housewives or harlots].[50] If they remained in the domestic sphere under the rule of father or husband, they ranked as honourable women. If entering the public sphere, the imputation of harlotry lingered, even if only as an atavistic threat. This dichotomy had ceased to function, if it ever had, in practical terms, but it remained part of the public consciousness. By the beginning of the twentieth century many French women had overthrown Proudhon's proscriptions by succeeding in public life. They nevertheless felt constrained not to undermine the ideal of female moral excellence by sexual unconventionality. As James F. McMillan argues though the *Belle Époque* saw significant advances for women's emancipation, counterbalancing this were fears, amounting to panic, at women's alleged defeminization.[51] To counter such alarms, women wishing to join the professions, to become teachers, doctors or lawyers, not only had to show their capacity to pass examinations and to demonstrate competence in their calling but, most importantly, to display moral

48 M.-H Renaut, 'Le droit et l'enfant adultérin de l'époque romaine à aujourd'hui', *Revue historique* (1997), 369–408.

49 Giroud, *FH*, 220.

50 For an analysis of Proudhon's significance for feminism see Georges Duby and Michelle Perrot, *Histoire des femmes: le XIX*e *siècle* (Paris: Plon, 1991), 74–76.

51 McMillan, *France and women*, 141–59.

probity – by which was meant, for women, chastity.[52] Not for them the liberating behaviour of 'les garçonnes' of the inter-war years.[53] Unmarried professional women should be 'irreproachable' in their morals. Those in the professions who did marry were especially lauded for their domestic roles.[54] Pascal who, given her medical training, was in no way a prude, was nevertheless sensitive to imputations of sexual laxity and had in the past resented family accusations that as a single woman in Paris she might have loose morals.[55] Above all, and quite apart from the general moral climate, she cannot have been unaware or untouched by the case of Marie Curie which had erupted in the press five years before.

One of the most famous scientists of her generation, Mme Curie was a byword for the highly talented woman who succeeds in a hitherto all-male profession.[56] She was an iconic model for ambitious women and had been singled out by Madeleine Pelletier in 1910 as an example of the cultural evolution of feminism. Like Pascal, Curie did not actively campaign as a feminist. Neither woman, by contrast to the notoriously militant and 'virile' Pelletier, challenged sexual stereotypes. They both seem to have thought that the avoidance of active militancy on the Pelletier model was the price of conquering their profession (Gordon, *IF*, 138–139).

Curie's public image was that of the tireless worker, the devoted wife and mother, and, when her husband Pierre Curie was killed in 1906, the inconsolable widow; all entirely genuine attributes. But she was also human, and by 1910, four years after her husband's death, had fallen deeply in love with a colleague, Professor Paul Langevin of the Collège de France, a married man with four children. When the story broke in the press in 1911, the same year that Marie Curie was

52 Margadant, *MLP*, 4.

53 Christine Bard, *Les Garçonnes: modes et fantasmes des années folles* (Paris: Flammarion, 1998). The term, 'les garçonnes' derives from a best-selling novel of the same name by Victor Margueritte (1922) which had a 'succès de scandale' by its depiction of the liberated sexual mores of his heroine but which ends with a return to conventional morality.

54 Anon, 'Femmes internes, hôpitaux et asiles', *La Vie heureuse* (February 1904), PRFP; Mary R. S. Creese, *Ladies in the Laboratory II: West European Women in Science, 1800–1900* (Lanham, Maryland and Oxford: The Scarecrow Press, 2004), 57–63; Marilyn B. Ogilvie, & J. Harvey, eds., *The Biographical Dictionary of Women in Science: Pioneering Lives from Ancient Times to the Mid-Twentieth-Century* (New York and London: Routledge, 2000), 403–04.

55 Corr CP & TP PRFP: n.d

56 See Françoise Giroud, *Une Femme honorable*, 207–15 and Marilyn B. Ogilvie, *Marie Curie: a biography* (Westport, CT and London: Greenwood Press, 2004).

awarded her second Nobel Prize, the scandal attained international proportions. Curie was vilified as a foreigner, a woman who had only succeeded through her husband, a home wrecker and, probably (in the right-wing press) a Jew. The affair stirred up a toxic mixture of misogyny, xenophobia and nationalism. Curie nearly lost her professorial post and would probably have done so had she been named as a co-respondent in the Langevin court case, finally settled, fortunately for her, by a formal separation rather than a divorce.[57] From a feminist perspective, Madeleine Pelletier was also outraged and did not mince her words:

> D'ailleurs comme vous le savez peut-être, Mme Curie prétend qu'elle n'est pas féministe. Son cas fera évidemment un très grand mal à notre cause; on dira, on dit, que pour la première fois que l'on fait une place à une femme, elle se conduit comme une catin. Elle aurait dû mettre de la discrétion dans ses relations avec le monsieur ; mais les femmes sont sans dignité. [...] Quand on aura émancipée l'amour, Mme Curie pourra coucher avec qui elle voudra, cela ne fera plus aucun tort au féminisme.[58]

> [Mme Curie claims that she is not a feminist. Her case will obviously do a great deal of damage to our cause; it will be said, it is being said, that the first time a place is made for a woman [in the highest academic circles] she behaves like a whore. She should have been more discreet in her relations with this gentleman; but women lack dignity. [...] When love has been emancipated, Mme Curie will be able to sleep with whoever she likes, this will no longer harm feminism.]

Even though Pascal was immured in the backwater of Clermont de l'Oise in 1911, she cannot but have been aware of the Curie-Langevin scandal and its implications for professional women generally. To suffer the public humiliation undergone by Curie, to risk losing her professional position and to endanger her daughter's future were fears that would haunt Pascal for the rest of her life.

In twenty-first-century Britain and France, where illegitimacy as a legal category has been abolished, it is difficult to appreciate the extent to which unmarried mothers were still viewed in the nineteenth and early twentieth centuries as being forever disgraced — as were their children. Pascal managed to retain her professional status and to care for and cherish her daughter, but not without making profound sacrifices. To account for the baby, Pascal fostered her as a war orphan, allegedly a victim of the conflict raging so close

57 Giroud, *FH*, 221–46.

58 Corr Pelletier-Ly, FMLB (13 November 1911).

to Clermont. Little Jeanne, was, as she had said in her journal, 'so late, but so much desired'. Her unfulfilled desire for a child must have haunted her youth. Though Pascal left no record of these earliest years with her daughter, two sources suggest some of her maternal preoccupations. The first is a letter written four years before the birth, in 1912, to her sister-in-law, Marie Pascal, detailing her theories of childcare; the second the series of bi-monthly articles on childcare, or périculture, that Pascal was commissioned to write in 1914–16 for *Le Petit Écho de la Mode*, a popular woman's magazine. Pascal's contacts with *Le Petit Écho* were due to her friends the Bouvard sisters, who managed the paper, had visited her at Clermont and who, as we have noted, were also friends of General Mengin.

To her sister-in-law, who must have complained of unhappiness in her marriage, Pascal commiserated, but urged that she was supremely fortunate to be the mother of her young son, Ion. She chided Marie for allowing her child to be brought up by servants:

> Permettez-moi de faire quelques réflexions sur votre vie. Vous n'êtes pas heureuse, je le sais. Je l'ai compris. Vous êtes trop intelligente pour trouver dans votre milieu des éléments de bonheur. Et pourtant vous en avez un tout près, en votre enfant. Pourquoi le laissez-vous avec votre horrible bonne ? À votre place, cet enfant serait à moi, à chaque heure du jour et de la nuit. Je ne voudrais pas de bonne et de gouvernante. C'est moi qui ferais tout pour lui. Je ne le quitterais pas une seconde. Cette vie si chère serait encore une fois pétrie de de ma vie. Comment supportez-vous qu'une étrangère vulgaire, dont vous ne voudriez pas à votre table, vive continuellement auprès de votre enfant et lui infuse ses sentiments, ses maigres idées. [...] Votre enfant ne doit pas vous quitter. Vous devez devenir son miroir et lui faire goûter, chaque jour, le lait de la tendresse humaine dont parle souvent Shakespeare (Corr CP & MP, PRFP, 8 September 1912).

> [Allow me to make some observations on your life. I know you are not happy. I understand that. You are too intelligent to find much happiness in your milieu. And yet you have a source of happiness beside you, in your child. Why do you leave him with your horrible maid? If I were in your place, this child would be with me at every hour of the day and night. I would not want a maid or a governess. I would do everything for him myself. I would not leave him for a second. This precious life would be once again filled with my life. How can you bear to allow a vulgar stranger, whom you would not allow to sit at your table, to live with your child and fill him with her sentiments and her petty ideas? [...] Your child should not leave your side. You should become his mirror and make him taste every day the milk of human kindness of which Shakespeare often speaks.]

Four years later, Pascal had the opportunity to put her theories into practice. The above letter suggests an overwhelming degree of devotion and attention to be focused on the child: 'Your child should not leave your side'. She was, of course writing to her Romanian sister-in-law, who lived in a gentrified culture, where most well-off people never dreamt of concerning themselves with the day-to-day care of their children. In Pascal's own case, her profession would force her to leave her child with child-minders for much of the day, but she exercised a high degree of care herself. The intensity of her maternal devotion might well have proved suffocating without the more indulgent influence of Justin Mengin and the resilient character, as it proved, of Jeanne Pascal herself. Little Jeanne always slept in her mother's room and was never away from her, except in a case of the latter's severe illness and once on a journey to England with her father in her teens. Pascal was determined to ensure that her daughter, born illegitimate, in a conservative Catholic culture where this still mattered very much, should not be handicapped by her birth. She supervised her daughter's health, her diet and especially her studies, where she showed herself a creative educator, especially in literature and the arts.

It was when she became a mother that Pascal began writing for *Le Petit Écho de la Mode*, owned since 1879 by a Catholic family from Brittany, a woman's magazine dedicated to the support of family values. Its pages were full of practical advice, combining the efficient running of the home with the spice of romance in the form of episodic novels. Emphasis was placed on women's duties rather than their rights. The huge success of this periodical, approved by the Church for its conservative Catholic morality and its endorsement of women's traditional role, points to the overriding importance of domestic ideology before, during and after the Great War.[59]

It is both poignant and ironic to think of this single mother writing for a journal that endorsed the most conservative social mores. The general heading for Pascal's articles was 'Les Devoirs d'une mère' [a mother's duties]. The sense of additional responsibilities for the family falling on women's shoulders, at a time when their husbands were away at war, permeates Pascal's medical advice on how to manage diet, exercise and childhood illnesses. 'Si, en temps de paix,

59 For the growth of a bourgeois or petit-bourgeois readership for women's magazines and their function in strengthening domestic ideology see Evelyn Sullerot, *La Presse féminine française* (Paris: Armand Colin, 1966), 7–59; Martine Bonvoisin Samra and Michèle Maignien, *La Presse féminine* (Paris: Presses Universitaires de France, 1986), 16; Christophe Charle, *Le Siècle de la presse, 1830–1939* (Paris: Seuil, 2004).

la vraie place de la femme est au foyer, en temps de guerre elle est partout où elle peut contribuer à la défense du pays' [Whereas, in times of peace, the women's true place is in the home, in times of war, her place is anywhere that she can contribute to the defence of her country].[60] From Constance Pascal, who railed against her brother for supposing that a woman's place was in the home and excoriated him for believing that her education should be commensurate with that destiny, this makes strange reading. But although she endorsed a 'woman's place', she also believed that the war had created new duties, roles and opportunities for women. By disseminating valuable medical information, her articles could be construed as 'contributing to the defence of her county'. Read as educational texts, they form an impressive series of informative documents on the nurture of children. In the course of writing them, Pascal was not only drawing on her medical knowledge of childhood illnesses, but was in practice engaged in caring for her own daughter. 'A mother's duties', as her articles were entitled, had become the central preoccupation of her life.

60 Constance Pascal 'La Protection des enfants', *Le Petit Écho de la mode* (25 March 1917).

4. Genius and Madness: Early Research and Writing, 1906–11

Pascal's successful viva for her doctoral thesis in 1905 was followed by the publication of at least ten scientific articles on early dementia and her monograph in 1911, *La Démence précoce* [*Dementia praecox*].[1] This research was undertaken during her posts as psychiatric intern at Ville Evrard under Paul Sérieux and at Perray Vaucluse. Subsequently as a *médecin adjoint* at Clermont de l'Oise, she drew on her clinical experience as well as on her wide reading in psychiatry, philosophy and the arts for her research which she pursued with passionate enthusiasm. As she would write to her Director in 1921, when applying for a new posting: 'Ce que je voudrais, c'est Strasbourg, c'est

1 Démence précoce was later to be termed schizophrenia; see Eugen Bleuler, 1908. The articles published by Constance Pascal in this period are: with Dr Courbon, 'Délire des préjudices préséniles' [Paranoid, schizophrenic mania], *L'Encéphale*, 2 (25 November 1906), 573–78. Single-authored articles: 'Formes prodromiques dépressives de la démence précoce' [Early depressive symptoms in *dementia praecox*], *Informateur des aliénistes et des neurologistes*, I (1906), 186–88; 'Les ictus dans la démence précoce' [Seizures in *dementia praecox*], *Informateur des aliénistes et des neurologistes*, II (1906), 139–44; 'La loi roumaine sur les aliénés: traduction et réflexions' [Romanian law concerning mental patients : translation and commentary], *Journal de médecine légale psychiatrique et d'anthropologie criminelle*, I (1906), 204–13; 'Le sourire et le rire dans la démence précoce'[Smiles and laughter in *dementia praecox*], *Journal de psychologie*, VI (1906), 392–407; 'Formes mélancoliques dans la démence précoce' [Melancholic forms of *dementia praecox*], *Archives de neurologie* (April 1907), 273–93; 'Les rémissions dans la démence précoce' [Remissions in *dementia praecox*], *Revue de psychiatrie* (April 1907), 147–61; 'Pseudo-neurasthénie prodromique de la démence précoce'[Pseudo-neurasthenic symptoms in *dementia praecox*], *La Presse médicale*, I (1907), 42–4; 'Les maladies mentales de Robert Schumann (génie et démence)' [The mental illnesses of Robert Schumann, genius and madness], *Journal de psychologie normale et pathologique*, 5 (1908), 98–130; 'La démence précoce: étude clinique et médico-légale'[*Dementia praecox*: clinical and medical-forensic study], *Revue de Médecine*, XXXI (1911), 304–33.

une mine d'or pour la recherche et le travail scientifique; c'est la seule chose qui m'intéresse ici-bas' [What I would like best is Strasbourg; it is a goldmine for research and scientific work, which are the only things that interest me in life].[2] This declaration, written when her daughter Jeanne, to whom she was devoted, was five years old, nevertheless underscores the emotional and intellectual divisions she imposed on herself. Her professional role and her family life remained rigorously separated.

'Research' in a psychiatric hospital at this time primarily involved the close observation of groups of patients, often chosen as objects of study in order to illustrate a particular condition and its variations. The titles of seven of Pascal's articles indicate the clinical observations on which they were based, for example: 'Formes prodromiques dépressives de la démence précoce' [Early depressive symptoms in *dementia praecox*]. A fictional representation of this clinical method can be found in Emile Zola's *L'Assommoir* (1877), an arresting picture of the final breakdown in alcoholism of his worker-protagonist Coupeau. Suffering from attacks of delirium tremens, this bellowing, screaming, incoherent, violently agitated creature in a padded cell at the Sainte Anne asylum in Paris is a caricature of what his wife Gervaise remembers:

> — Seigneur! qu'est-ce qu'il a donc?... qu'est-ce qu'il a donc?... répétait Gervaise, prise de taf. Un interne, un gros garçon blond et rose, en tablier blanc, tranquillement assis, prenait des notes. Le cas était curieux, l'interne ne quittait pas le malade.[3]
>
> [Good Lord! What's the matter with him, what's the matter with him? said Gervaise, scared stiff. A [psychiatric] house physician, a big, fair, rosy-cheeked young man in a white coat, was sitting there calmly taking notes. It was a fascinating case and he never left the patient's side.]

Without querying scientific objectivity, which was, after all, the method he claimed to employ in his fiction, Zola underscores the contrast between the doctor, pleased to find such an excellent example of delirium tremens to study, and Coupeau, the victim of alcohol poisoning, undergoing the tortures of the damned, who has become the unwitting object of professional observation and psychiatric

2 Corr CP & Dir, Prémontré DACP (16 September 1921).

3 Emile Zola, *L'Assommoir* (1877) (Paris: Fasquelle, 1962), 485; Emile Zola, *L'Assommoir* (Harmondsworth: Penguin, 1970), 409.

interest.[4] Nor does Gervaise's horrified response to her husband's condition find any sympathetic echo in the young man calmly taking notes. Like Zola, Constance Pascal begins to suggest in her early psychiatric writing that the problem of 'objective' knowledge for psychiatrists is that its pursuit can cancel out the perception of a patient's real suffering and the reality of his or her feelings.

It is probable that Pascal was able to specialize in *dementia praecox* in part thanks to her fluent German, which must have proved a boon to her supervisor, Dr Paul Sérieux, in disseminating the theories of the leading German psychiatrist in the subject, Emil Kraepelin (1856–1926). Pascal corresponded with Kraepelin, who even suggested she might collaborate with him. As women had been admitted to the medical profession in Prussia after 1890, Kraepelin seems to have been happy to welcome another female researcher into his field:[5]

> Sehr geehrtes Fräulein!
>
> Auf Ihr freundliches Schreiben beehre ich mich, zu erwidern, dass ich zur Zeit leider nicht in der Lage bin, Ihnen irgend etwas Neues über meine Auffassung der *Dementia praecox* sagen zu können. Selbstverständlich habe ich im Laufe der letzten Jahre auch allerlei neue Erfahrungen gesammelt und meine früheren Anschauungen nach manchen Richtungen hin berichtigt. Allein zu einer planmässigen Durcharbeitung der ganzen Frage bin ich noch nicht gekommen, da ich durch die Neuauflage meiner allgemeinen Psychiatrie zu sehr in Anspruch genommen war. Erst jetzt, wo diese Arbeit beendet ist, werde ich mich wieder mehr mit klinischen Fragen beschäftigen können. Ich möchte Sie aber nicht durch voreilige und nur auf allgemeine Eindrücke sich stützende Meinungen beeinflussen, bevor es mir nicht [*sic*] möglich gewesen ist, mein großes klinisches Material selbst wieder einmal gründlich durchzuarbeiten. Ich hoffe aber lebhaft, dass die von Ihnen in Aussicht gestellten Studien mir auch für meine Arbeit wertvolle Förderung bringen werden; in etwa Jahresfrist gedenke ich fertig zu werden. Wollen Sie einmal bei uns arbeiten, so werden Sie uns stets willkommen sein.
>
> In collegialer Hochachtung verbleibe ich Ihr ganz ergebener,
>
> Kraepelin[6]

4 In 'Le Roman experimental' [The Experimental Novel], 1880, Zola developed his theory of scientific realism in fiction referred to as naturalism. Zola himself was the object of a psychological study by Édouard Toulouse in 1896, see Michel Huteau, *Psychologie, psychiatrie et société sous la Troisième République: la biocratie d'Édouard Toulouse (1865–1947)* (Paris: Harmattan, 2002), 67–75.

5 Richard J. Evans, *The Feminists* (London: Croom Helm, 1977), 111–12.

6 Corr Emil Kraepelin & CP, PRFP (26 May 1909).

> [Dear Mademoiselle
>
> I have the honour of replying to your kind letter; but I must tell you that unfortunately I am unable at the moment to offer you any new information on my conception of *dementia praecox*. Of course in the last few years I have accumulated many new observations and taken my earlier findings in various new, more accurate directions. However I have not yet been able to achieve a fully coherent treatment of the whole question, as I have been too busy with the revision of my general psychiatry book. Now that this work is finished, I will be able to spend more time on clinical questions. I would not wish to influence you with opinions based on over-hasty or general impressions before I have had the chance to go through my extensive clinical material again. I have every confidence and hope, however, that the studies you are proposing will also bring valuable improvements to my work, which I expect to complete in around one year. If at any time you wish to work with us, you will always be welcome.
>
> With collegial esteem I remain your devoted,
>
> Kraepelin]

Though he issued a cautionary warning that she should not put too much weight on his unfinished research, the fact that one of the most influential psychiatrists in Europe invited Pascal to collaborate was a signal honour. While much of the French scientific climate was hostile to German ideas, a legacy of the French defeat in the Franco-Prussian War, Pascal's contacts with Kraepelin demonstrate that she was actively engaged with German-language research in psychiatry. She had read Jung and Freud at least a decade before they were translated into French, or were widely made known to a French public.[7] Recalling the anti-German remarks in her War Journal, however, it is clear that her interest in German psychiatry, like her wide reading in German philosophy and literature, was secondary to her love of France. Her adopted country had become and remained her spiritual and intellectual home.

Kraepelin, whose theories underpinned Pascal's clinical observations, had assumed a medical model for mental disorders.[8]

7 Translations of Freud's work did not appear in France until 1922, with Jankélévitch's translations. For a discussion of Freud's reception in France see Elisabeth Roudinesco, *La Bataille de cent ans: histoire de la psychanalyse en* France (Paris: Ramsay, vol. 1: Seuil, vol. 2, 1982–86); Jacques Postel and Claude Quétel, *Nouvelle Histoire de la psychiatrie* (Paris: Dunod, 1983); Sherry Turkle, *Psychoanalytic Politics: Freud's French Revolution* (London: Deutsch, 1979) and Ohayon, *L'Impossible Rencontre* (1999).

8 Emil Kraepelin, *Dementia praecox and paraphrenia*, trans. by Mary Barclay from the eighth German edition, ed. George M. Robertson (Edinburgh: Livingstone, 1919).

His work was largely nosological, undertaking the systematic classification of diseases, based on the cause, course and termination of each disease. Mental illness was held to have an organic basis.[9] His system brought greater consistency to psychiatric classification, allowing clinicians to compare the same phenomena in different patients and hospitals. He described *dementia praecox* as having three forms or states: hebephrenic, catatonic and paranoid.[10] Kraepelin's medical model of the organic origins of mental disorder resembled Pierre Janet's degeneracy theory, in the sense that mental illness was deemed inevitable in certain individuals and therapeutic intervention of little use. The emphasis on classification to the near exclusion of therapeutic methods became the staple method of early twentieth-century psychiatry. In reading Pascal's application of Kraepelin's theories we see this nosological limitation in her discussions. More original are glimpses of her interest in the emotional and imaginative side of her patients' minds. Diagnostic precision or semiology, the reading of signs, was not enough. In her view:

> En psychiatrie particulièrement, les données de nos observations sont trop incomplètes pour qu'on trouve celle qui révèle la qualité principale. En outre, la signification et la vérité scientifiques ne résident pas seulement dans la clarté des faits, mais dans la pénombre et les perspectives fuyantes qui les environnent.[11]

> [In psychiatry especially, the data available to us are too incomplete to discover the key one which will reveal the principal quality of an illness. Furthermore, meaning and scientific truth are to be found there not only in clearly established facts but in the half-light and vanishing perspectives that surround them.]

The condition of *dementia praecox*, also known as youthful madness, had been known since antiquity. Its cause was much disputed. Was it organic, i.e. physical, or a purely mental/psychic disorder? Studies

9 John C. Burnham, 'Kraepelin, Emil (1856–1926)' in *International Encyclopaedia of Psychiatry, Psychology, Psychoanalysis and Neurology*, IX (New York: Aesculapius, 1997) considers Kraepelin a successful synthesizer of psychiatric theory by charting the prognosis of a given disease. Kraepelin convincingly identified two 'endogenous' disease processes, *dementia praecox* and manic-depressive insanity. Assuming a constitutional predisposition to mental illness, he dissented from the prevailing theory of degeneracy, particularly prevalent in France. Kraepelin's model, however, did not lend itself to developing treatments for mental illness.

10 Hebrephrenia, the 'madness of youth', is a sub-type of what is now called schizophrenia, showing marked disorganization of speech and behaviour, inappropriate affect and unsystematic and bizarre delusions.

11 Pascal, *La Démence précoce*, quoted in Barbier, *VOCP*, 79.

of syphilitic patients with what was termed general paralysis (the subject of Pascal's doctoral thesis) and the terminal development of that disease strengthened the case, it was thought, for a physical origin for other psychiatric conditions such as *dementia praecox*.[12] It was assumed that the brains of affected patients carried toxic lesions. Like her contemporaries, therefore, Pascal assumed an organic cause.

Prior to Kraepelin's work, B.A. Morel (1809–73), who first coined the term, had tied *dementia praecox* to degeneracy theory. Morel's conception of *dementia praecox* identified two 'precocious aspects' of the condition: early onset (often during puberty) and rapid development into full dementia with the intellect terminally weakened. Kraepelin's reading of *dementia praecox*, by contrast, made a distinction between curable and incurable cases, suggesting the possibility of remission or even cure. Nevertheless, in the seventh edition of his *Treatise on dementia praecox* (1904), the one Pascal probably consulted, the illness was identified as a condition evolving towards almost complete mental disorganization. Causation was assumed to be genital in origin and triggered by puberty. Kraepelin's theories were, as we have seen, championed by Paul Sérieux in France, who wrote his own *La Démence précoce* in 1902, followed by Masselon in 1904, with a work with the same title. While Constance believed there were hereditary factors to dementia, she did not see this as a sufficient explanation for the onset of illness. Her monograph, *La Démence précoce* of 1911, would be a definitive summation of the condition and remained the authoritative work on it until the 1950s.[13] Concurrently, however, Kraepelin's model of *dementia praecox* was absorbed into the category schizophrenia, as defined by Bleuler, who published his treatise on the subject in 1911, the same year that Pascal's book appeared. Her subsequent neglect in the history of psychiatry can partly be explained by the fact that her major theoretical work was tied to a disappearing classification.

In her clinical observations of *dementia praecox*, published between 1906 and 1909, based on Kraepelin's classification, Pascal focused on the importance of early and correct diagnosis and the need to distinguish between *dementia praecox* and depression or neurasthenia. She noted, as Bleuler would later, the lack of coordination between

12 For a discussion of the identification of the syphilis microbe and the identification of general paralysis as being a tertiary and final stage of syphilitic infection see Claude Quétel, *History of Syphilis* [Le Mal de Naples: historie de la syphilis] (1986) trans. by Judith Braddock and Brian Pike (London: Polity Press, 1993), 139–75.

13 Barbier, *VOCP*, 77; Corr Professor H. Baruk & Jeanne Pascal Rees, PRFP (27 October 1968).

an ostensible response shown by a patient (laughter for example) and underlying unhappiness. This disorganized state of affectivity represented, she suggested, one of the most telling symptoms of the illness. When analysing seizures in patients, she made the case for distinguishing between epilepsy, *dementia praecox* and general paralysis.[14] A further semiological distinction followed in her article on melancholic symptoms in patients, which could indicate either depression or *dementia praecox*. In depression Pascal looked for a precipitating trauma to trigger the illness, whereas *dementia praecox* could appear without any precipitating event.[15] While following and expounding Kraepelin's theories, Pascal began to develop her own. For example, in 'Les rémissions dans la démence précoce' (1907) [Remissions in *dementia praecox*], while remaining wedded to the idea of the organic origin of the disease, she argued that some cases showed such marked remission that one could speak of cure. She focused also on the psychological aspect of the illness – an early indication of an interest she would develop later in her career. She noted the existence of emotional regression in the early stages, even though the patient was still able to reason and to understand general ideas. In the second and final stage this conceptual element too disappeared. Remission, she believed, was possible only in the first stage.

Pascal's early works show an evolution from a purely organicist position to a psycho-biological reading of the thought disorders associated with *dementia praecox*. Fundamentally, she retained Kraepelin's assumptions but, in the context of early twentieth-century French psychiatry, showed considerable originality by illustrating their value in clinical diagnosis. Pascal's research was necessarily determined by her professional context, in that her articles rested on the observation and semiological definition of various symptoms. At the same time she began to articulate her characteristic involvement and sympathy with her patients, noting how their emotions affected their reasoning processes.

Two of Pascal's articles at this period, 'Les ictus dans la démence précoce' [Seizures in *dementia praecox*] (1906) and 'Les Maladies mentales de Robert Schumann' [The mental illnesses of Robert Schumann] (1908) are of particular interest as illustrating her empirical method, scholarly reading and wider humanist or cultural concerns. The basic psycho-medical premise of 'Seizures', that the illness is caused by toxins creating lesions in the brain which effect the sensory, but not the motor, zones of activity, has largely historical

14 'Formes prodromiques dépressives de la démence précoce' (1906).

15 'Formes mélancoliques dans la démence précoce' (1907).

interest. Pascal sought to classify and thereby to understand seizures and convulsions as an indication of the early stages of *dementia praecox* and to distinguish them from those of epileptics and hysterics. The question she attempted to answer was: are convulsions in patients a parallel affliction to *dementia praecox*, or are they an early indication of a later, still developing condition? In marshalling her evidence, Pascal demonstrated an impressive range of medical and psychiatric references in three languages – French, German and English. The article constituted a review of the existing literature on the subject, in which she did not hesitate to dispute the conclusions of some experts in the field, notably Reynaud, Charcot and Janet. She concluded that in genuine cases of hysteria and epilepsy, dating from childhood, these might exist in association with *dementia praecox*, but there was also strong evidence that there were seizures belonging specifically to *dementia praecox*, which were not separate hysterical or epileptic symptoms.

'Seizures in *dementia praecox*' illustrates Pascal's clarity of argument, her elegant style in a language which was not her mother-tongue, the range of her medical-psychiatric reading, her intellectual and professional confidence and her authority over her subject. The conclusions, based on a biological-pathological model, accurately reflected the state of biomedical science of the day. She insisted on close clinical observation of signs and symptoms, convinced that the meaning of the patients' seizures, hallucinations and indeed silences lay at the heart of the mystery of mental illness, the possible clues as to their mental life. The labels affixed to mental disorders, though diagnostically useful, did not replicate the affective reality of those disorders.

Whereas Pascal's diagnostic and classificatory psychiatric work demonstrated her professional engagement and competence, her analysis of the composer Robert Schumann (1810–56) and his history of mental illness is of wider cultural interest. Like Maupassant, Van Gogh, Dostoevsky and other nineteenth-century artists, Schumann's mental afflictions received, and continued to receive, a great deal of scrutiny from scholars, as well as from mental health professionals.[16] A well-documented patient during his lifetime, Schumann also left diaries and correspondence offering insights into his illness. Pascal's

16 There is a wide range of biographical literature on Schumann. See for example: Victor Basch, *Schumann: a Life of Suffering*, trans. C. A. Phillips (New York: Alfred A. Knopf, 1928); Peter Ostwald, *Schumann: Music and Madness* (London: Victor Gollancz, 1985); Rémy Stricker, *Robert Schumann: le musicien et la folie* (Paris: Gallimard, 1984); Robert Taylor, *Robert Schumann: His Life and Work* (London: Granada, 1982).

choice of title for her article, using the plural (The mental illnesses of Robert Schumann), contributed to the long-standing debate about Schumann's madness and expanded a theme, previously developed in her 'Seizures', of the possibility of distinct mental illnesses existing in the same individual over time.

Apart from her professional psychiatric interest, Pascal studied Schumann's mental breakdowns because it gave her the opportunity to examine the issue of genius and madness, as theorized by Cesare Lombroso.[17] Was madness a sign of genius, or alternatively were all geniuses insane, or potentially insane? Through her Schumann study, Pascal was concerned to refute Lombroso's identification of genius with madness. Her approach to Schumann's condition was initially nosological – the difficulty would be to classify the known empirical signs of his mental disturbances to find the most likely diagnostic category. In this vein, the article opens with a robust defence of the value of psychological enquiry into the mentality of men of genius:

> Quelques littérateurs se sont révoltés contre les médecins et psychologues qui étudient la mentalité des grands hommes et osent mettre une étiquette sur leurs souffrances physiques et morales. [...] L'histoire de la vie d'un homme de génie est une page de l'histoire de la pensée humaine, elle ne doit être indifférente à personne. [...] L'esprit d'un homme de génie est soumis aux mêmes lois que le terrain biologique sur lequel il repose. [...] Étudier scientifiquement un homme de génie, c'est briser les murailles dans lesquelles on enferme les mystères de la nature, c'est jeter quelques lueurs sur les lois et les destinées de la vie de l'homme ('Schumann', 98–99).
>
> [Some literary hacks are outraged by doctors and psychologists who study the mentality of great men and dare to put a label on their physical and mental sufferings. [...] The history of a genius's life is a page in the history of human thought and should not be a matter of indifference to anyone. [...] The mind of a genius is subject to the same laws as the biological ground on which he stands. [...] To study a genius scientifically is to break down the walls that shut away the mysteries of nature; it can cast a few glimmers of light on the laws and destinies of human life.]

Arguing that the power of genius was not diminished by a scientific understanding of an individual's mental strengths and weaknesses, Pascal asserted that all minds, however exceptional, are ruled by their biological makeup. The creative drive was a product not of mind or spirit but, as Sainte-Beuve had said, of blood and

17 See Cesare Lombroso, *L'Homme de génie* [*L'uomo di genio in rapporto alla psichiatria*] (1888), trans. Colona d'Istria (Paris: Alcan, 1909).

muscle.[18] Nevertheless, a psychiatric label was only the first step in understanding the human mind. Thus a mental map or analysis of Robert Schumann's condition would require different levels of understanding, involving observations based on psycho-physiology and pathology, and ranging beyond these to philosophy and music criticism.

Pascal emphasized both Schumann's genius and the extent to which his illness was the cause of genuine suffering:

> Cet homme prodigieux était un malade. De l'âge de vingt-trois ans à celui de quarante-six auquel il mourut, il ne passa pas beaucoup de jours sans souffrir. Son mal était toujours à ses côtés comme un ennemi. Toute sa vie n'a été qu'une lutte à mort sans relâche et sans trêve entre les deux forces, celle du génie qui se défend, s'affirme et s'épanouit, et celle de la maladie qui envahit, ronge et détruit petit à petit son âme et son corps. [...] Schumann éternisa ses souffrances par son œuvre étrange et sublime. Ses cris de détresse ont répandu sur les sentiers du monde la semence de la douleur et créèrent des sources infinies d'émotions ('Schumann', 99).
>
> [This prodigious man was ill. From the age of twenty-three to forty-six, when he died, he spent very few days without suffering. His illness was always at his side like an enemy. His whole life was nothing but a battle to the death, without respite and or truce, between two powers, that of his genius affirming, flourishing and defending itself, and that of his illness which was invading, undermining and destroying him, body and soul. Through his strange and sublime music Schumann immortalized his suffering. His cries of distress sowed the seeds of pain all over the world and created infinite wellsprings of emotion.]

His music, she believed, was a record of his torment, which is why an understanding of his sensibility and its pathological manifestations were so important. Through his ability to convey profound emotion in music, with the transforming power of genius, Schumann changed our perception of reality. Was this the genius of madness, or genius responding with insight to periodic mental instability?

Since direct observation of the patient was impossible, Pascal reviewed the previous theories of Schumann's illness before outlining a clinical picture based on biographical and autobiographical sources. An autopsy of his brain done at the time of Schumann's death in 1856 by Dr Richards at the Endenich Asylum near Bonn, where the composer was interned, which supposedly revealed some lesions, was now thought to be unreliable. Richard's report had fuelled the

18 Charles-Augustin Sainte-Beuve (1804–69); French poet, novelist and major literary critic.

theory proposed by Wassentensky that Schumann suffered from degeneracy of the brain. Then in 1894, thirty-eight years after his death, Schumann's skull was examined by a Dr Schauffhausen who made a craniometrical analysis of his head and brain. Craniometry assumed that the size and capacity of the skull indicated the intellectual capacity of an individual.[19] But since by 1908 craniometry had been discredited as a pseudo-science, this study too had little value. In 1906 Möbius had published a developmental study of Schumann's mental illness and diagnosed *dementia praecox*. Möbius's diagnosis in its turn was refuted by a Dr Grüle of Heidelberg, who thought Schumann suffered from a manic-depressive psychosis complicated by terminal brain changes. Thus in her literature review of Schumann's illness, Pascal underscored the still-open debate on Schumann's illness before embarking on her 'clinical observation'.

The details of Schumann's biography are well known. What follows is a selection of data Pascal chose to inform her psychiatric diagnosis. She began with heredity. Schumann's father, an intelligent and cultivated man, had shown a tendency to melancholia. His mother, also intelligent, was characterized as highly emotional. Schumann's three brothers and one sister all died young, the sister after a prolonged mental illness, possibly *dementia praecox*. Schumann had a troubled adolescence, manifesting excessive sensibility. Both music and Romantic literature could throw him into crises of pathological nervousness. His musical genius surfaced relatively late. His hopes of becoming a concert pianist were aborted by problems with one finger of his right hand. The origin and extent of this injury and whether it was self-inflicted are still a matter of dispute among biographers. The death in 1833 of his sister-in-law, to whom he was devoted, seems to have precipitated attacks of vertigo. Schumann began to fear that he was losing his reason. His marriage in 1840 to Clara Wieck, the gifted concert pianist, ushered in a short period of happiness and productivity, though fears of death and madness, while acting as a spur to his musical expression, continued to haunt him. The next ten years were a period of great creativity, punctuated by mental crises, phobias, obsessions and auditory hallucinations. Nevertheless, in spite of these episodes, according to Pascal, his intellect was unaffected.

19 For background on craniometry see Robert Young, *Mind, Brain and Adaptation in the Nineteenth Century* (Oxford: Oxford University Press, 1970); Theodore Zeldin, *France 1848–1945: vol. 2* (Oxford: Oxford University Press, 1970), 774–79; Elizabeth Fee, 'Nineteenth-century craniology: the study of the female skull', *Bulletin of the History of Medicine*, 53 (1979), 423–33; Stephen Jay Gould, *The Mismeasure of Man* (London: Norton, 1981).

Between 1845 and 1850, Schumann composed at least thirty major works. Exhaustion, however, took its toll and in 1850 he began to experience more serious mental disturbances. By 1852 convulsive attacks had set in, inaugurating a period of rapid decline. Pascal detailed a chronology of Schumann's increasing distress and hallucinations culminating in a suicide attempt on 27 February 1854, when he threw himself into the river. Following his rescue, he was interned at the Endennich Asylum. In 1855 some improvement in his mental state was reported, but this proved temporary. He refused food and seems to have starved himself to death, dying in 1856 at the age of forty-six.

From these reported clinical observations Pascal concluded that from the age of twenty-one to forty-one Schumann suffered from a constitutional illness, physical in origin and probably hereditary. She believed this to be a psycho-neurosis, a disturbance not qualified as madness or dementia. She dissented from the views of Dr Richards who thought that Schumann suffered throughout his adult life from general paralysis and melancholia, a progressive disease, and from Möbius's opinion that he had *dementia praecox* in an intermediary form. Pascal argued that from the age of forty-one a different illness overtook him, which took a progressive and fatal form. In her view, the earlier neurosis and the latter disorder were separate phenomena.

Pascal's grounds for taking issue with the diagnosis of *dementia praecox*, in which, of course she had specialized, were Schumann's 'mutisme', his long periods of silence, which she denied were pathological. Schumann, she suggested, simply liked quiet; silence was a necessary condition for creativity. Further, though he suffered from hallucinations for many years, he did not deteriorate mentally until the last two or three years of his life. Nor did Pascal accept the diagnosis of manic depression. Schumann, she argued, was never manic, though often depressed. While agreeing that there could never be an absolute diagnosis, she believed that he initially suffered from pyschasthenia, a term coined by Pierre Janet, to denote a neurosis characterized by anxiety, doubt and indecision, with an impulse to perfectionism, accompanied by inhibitions, feelings of impotence and rapid fatigue.[20]

20 Pierre Janet (1859–1947) was a disciple of Charcot, who appointed him director of the psychiatric laboratory at the Salpêtrière in Paris. In 1904 he founded the *Journal de psychologie normale et pathologique*. Janet classified the neuroses: hysteria, caused by failure of personality integration and psychasthenia, which resulted from a general lowering of nervous tension.

One of the questions behind the attempt to diagnose Schumann's condition was the issue of general paralysis. Among the most common psychiatric diagnoses of the late nineteenth and early twentieth centuries, the term fell out of use when it became clear that the condition represented the tertiary stages of syphilis, although the link was not definitively established until 1913.[21] By 1908, when Pascal published her article, the association of general paralysis with the final stages of the disease was still being resisted by the French psychiatric establishment, though already in 1907 Plaut had obtained positive results from the recently perfected Bordet-Wassermann test, and found syphilis in patients suffering from general paralysis. Though she does not speak of syphilis in her Schumann article, Pascal would certainly have known of the debate surrounding the condition and its presumed connections to general paralysis. In this case, rejecting the diagnosis of *dementia praecox*, which she believed would not have allowed Schumann's mental faculties to flower as they did, she argued that in spite of repeated nervous crises, he was, when composing music, entirely sane. In relation to his psychiatric profile after 1850, on the other hand, she opted for the concept of a further illness, probably general paralysis, with all that this might imply of a syphilitic infection.

Pascal's reading of Schumann's mental illnesses can be understood not only in the context of psychiatric diagnoses, but more significantly in relation to medical and cultural definitions of genius, madness and greatness. Schumann provided a valuable case history to test the concept of genius itself and the question of whether it was not only allied to, but even a product of, madness. In describing Schumann's final collapse, after he had been forced to resign his post as conductor at Düsseldorf, Pascal tellingly evokes Nietzsche, another genius-victim of syphilis:

> Pour l'esprit comme pour le corps, cesser de travailler, c'est commencer à mourir. Le Génie du son éteint sa torche. Une maladie terrible, qui ne pardonne pas, lui enleva progressivement toutes ses facultés: sa volonté, son intelligence, sa sensibilité exquise, source intarissable de tant de belles créations artistiques. Il disparut comme le surhomme de Nietzsche 'au moment où il a atteint le suprême degré de la sagesse, au moment où le soleil de son existence est au zénith, à l'heure du « grand midi », en consacrant par sa mort, le triomphe de sa doctrine' ('Schumann', 113).
>
> [For the mind, just as for the body, to give up work is to begin to die. This genius of sound was putting out his flame. A terrible, fatal illness

21 Quétel, *Syphilis*, 139–75.

> [*the onset of terminal, tertiary syphilis*] robbed him progressively of all his faculties: his willpower, his intelligence, his exquisite sensibility, the unquenchable source of so many beautiful artistic creations. He vanished like Nietzsche's superman 'at the moment when he had attained the highest degree of wisdom, at the moment when the sun of his existence was at its zenith, at "high noon", consecrating by his death the triumph of his doctrine'.]

Pascal had read and admired the philosopher's ideas on exceptional individuals, identifying her own drive and ambition with the figure of Nietzsche's superman. Her War Journal refers repeatedly to genius battling mediocrity. Drawing on the parallels between Schumann and Nietzsche, Pascal read Schumann's illness as paradigmatic of gifted individuals whose nervous constitutions could destroy them. For Pascal, it was of overriding importance to establish the sanity of genius, to demonstrate that the highly gifted individual could escape from the prison of mental torment to reach his fellow men through the power of art. The masculine gender is hers: she does not tackle the question as to whether only men were geniuses, as did her contemporary, Madeleine Pelletier.[22] Implicitly, however, she aligns herself with Nietzsche's model of individualism.

In 1911 Pascal published a condensed version of her much longer monograph on *dementia praecox* in the *Revue de Médecine,* summarising her work in the field.[23] It dealt with the history, nosology, symptoms, characteristic mental weaknesses, development, organic basis, possible causal factors, pathology, diagnosis, relevance to legal medicine and (briefly) treatment of the disease. Intriguingly, this study marked her first tentative engagement with Freud and Jung. Her primary aim was to demonstrate that *dementia praecox,* which can strike in all social classes and both sexes, and particularly the young, was as important in mental medicine as general paralysis of the insane. The variety of symptoms in *dementia praecox* made it a rewarding though difficult field for psychological study:

> L'apparition fréquente de la démence précoce pendant la période des études (enfance, puberté, adolescence), expose les éducateurs à de nombreuses méprises. La plupart de ces jeunes malades son confondus avec les enfants anormaux ou considérés comme des vicieux, mal élevés, paresseux, entêtés etc., et deviennent l'objet de corrections et de peines disciplinaires. Souvent, la démence précoce s'attaque à ces

22 Madeleine Pelletier, 'Les Femmes peuvent-elles avoir du génie?' (Paris, *c.* 1905), BMD.

23 Constance Pascal, 'La démence précoce: (étude clinique et médico-légale)', *Revue de médecine,* XXXI (1911), 304–33.

élèves brillants qui font l'orgueil des parents. Après avoir donné les signes d'une intelligence pleine de promesses, ils n'apprennent plus rien; ils deviennent incapables d'évoluer, d'acquérir des connaissances nouvelles et de se plier à un travail régulier ('Démence', 304–5).

[The frequent appearance of *dementia praecox* during the years of study (childhood, puberty, adolescence) leads educators into many errors. Most of these young patients are mistaken for children with abnormalities, or considered to be depraved, badly behaved, lazy, stubborn etc., and thus subjected to punishments and disciplinary sanctions. *Dementia praecox* often attacks brilliant pupils, who are the pride of their parents. After showing exceptional intellectual promise, they suddenly stop learning, appear incapable of further development or of acquiring new knowledge and seem unable to work in a disciplined way.]

Pascal was particularly interested in the social dimension of the disease. Many young people, who had engaged in criminal acts resulting in a prison sentence, were in fact suffering from a mental illness. The early signs of *dementia praecox* needed to be better understood by doctors and magistrates. She invoked the key role that Kraepelin had played in identifying the syndrome:

C'est à Kræpelin (1899) que revient l'honneur d'avoir groupé en une entité morbide les démences vésaniques et un grand nombre d'états dépressifs, maniaques, confusionnels, stuporeux, hystériformes, délirants polymorphes ou mal systématisés qui ne trouvaient place dans aucun cadre précis. Le mérite du professeur de Munich est d'avoir démontré que ces états morbides, en apparence distincts, ont la même évolution et le même pronostic, le même mode de début et de terminaison et qu'ils sont les manifestations aiguës d'un affaiblissement mental spécial: *la démence précoce* ('Démence', 305–6).

[We are indebted to Kraepelin (1899) for having grouped together as one pathological entity those chronic mental disorders and a large number of depressive, manic, confusional, catatonic, hysterical, polymorphous deliria, which had not been systematically defined or put in any clear framework. It is to the great credit of this Munich professor that he has shown how these seemingly distinct morbid states have the same aetiology and the same prognosis, the same way of beginning and ending, and that they are the acute signs of a particular mental deterioration, *dementia praecox*.]

Kraepelin had not merely gathered a heterogeneous group of mental and physical symptoms and put them under one rubric, he had proved convincingly that these multitudinous signs of mental disturbance belonged to a single illness because their origin and trajectory were so similar.

In her literature review, Pascal summarizes debates over the symptoms and development of *dementia praecox*. The essential characteristics of the illness are (a) a toxic process, organic in origin, which degrades brain tissue; (b) an attack on young people, appearing often in puberty or adolescence; (c) a mental deterioration, especially marked by the destruction of affective impulses. 'L'être sentant disparaît avant l'être pensant' ('Démence', 308) [The feeling individual disappears before the thinking individual]. Particularly significant in Pascal's view was this weakening of feelings, first noted by Kraepelin who had written:

> L'indifférence des malades à l'égard de leurs affections d'autrefois, notamment la disparition des sentiments pour la famille, les amis, etc., sont très souvent le premier et le meilleur signe du début de l'affection. Même si les mouvements expressifs sont vivaces, les malades ne sentent aucune joie véritable, aucune tristesse, ne conservent ni désirs, ni répugnances, vivent indifférents au jour le jour. ('Démence', 308–9.)
>
> [The indifference of patients towards those whom they used to love, especially the disappearance of family feeling and friendship, is very often the first and clearest sign of the onset of the illness. Even if they exhibit strong emotion, the patients feel no real joy or sadness, retain no desires or dislikes, and their lives drift along in a state of indifference.]

Not only, remarked Pascal, do patients lose family, moral and social feelings; they also experience a diminution in their own personality, a weakening of the ego. This inability to concentrate on or experience feelings leads patients to leave their normal occupations, become isolated and plunge into a physical and moral inertia.

After detailing the effects of *dementia praecox* on the patient's attitudes (negativism), gestures (often wild and uncoordinated), language (increasingly incoherent), Pascal traces the evolution of the illness, laying particular emphasis on the premonitory or prodromic period, followed by the active and then residual stage. The first diagnosis, because it could be confused with other mental disorders, e.g. hysteria, was the most difficult. Patients in this early stage were aware of losing their unified personality; the outside world, memories, perceptions and ideas became increasingly imprecise. Tell-tale signs of the illness such as tics, explosive laughter, grimaces, eccentricities and opinionated views combined with exaggerated docility all revealed the advent of mental disorder. There were cases of unexplained remission, sometimes of a few months only, but occasionally for long periods and to a degree that amounted to cure. Pursuing the question of aetiology, or causation, Pascal raised the comparison with general paralysis and made it clear that she was a partisan of the Wassermann test for syphilis, indicated as a new discovery, 'qui sera de la plus grande utilité diagnostique' [which will be extremely useful in diagnosis]. In welcoming the Wassermann test as a diagnostic tool, Pascal was in advance of much of her profession.

The section on 'Forensic Medicine' deals with the early stages of *dementia praecox*, when sufferers might begin to act bizarrely or fall into criminal behaviour. Pascal had a long-standing interest in the relationship between anti-social actions and mental illness and felt that many juvenile offenders, in particular, should not be imprisoned but given medical-psychiatric treatment. Nevertheless, treatment was certainly problematic, given the supposed organic basis of the illness. Apart from experimental and heroic interventions carried out by a number of psychiatrists – thyroid injections or, alternatively, removal of the thyroid; lumbar punctures or, most strangely, giving goat's serum infected with the blood of a catatonic patient – so-called medical treatments produced only the most modest benefits, if any at all. More efficacious in Pascal's view was productive labour, especially gardening. In an age when able-bodied mental patients were expected to work for their board in asylums, she observed the therapeutic value of being engaged in meaningful activity, a realisation still acted upon today through occupational therapy schemes.

On the question of the possible prevention of *dementia praecox*, Pascal offers a disappointingly moralistic answer:

> Le traitement préventif de la démence précoce est celui de toutes les psychoses. Il consiste dans l'application des règles de l'hygiène et dans l'éducation morale. [...] L'éducation morale a pour but d'apprendre aux jeunes gens à résister aux impulsions et aux tentations, de développer les sentiments de justice, de solidarité et le sens moral ('Démence', 333).
>
> [The preventative treatment of *dementia praecox* is the same as for all psychoses. It consists in the application of the rules of hygiene and in a moral education. [...] The aim of moral education is to teach young people to resist their impulses and temptations and to develop their feelings of justice, solidarity and morality.]

One wonders how even a coercive educational and social indoctrination could spare individuals the horrors of *dementia praecox*, which Pascal, like her psychiatric peers, believed had a physical, not a psychological basis. Since it was argued that the affective aspect of personality, closely allied to the moral sense, disappeared in the early stages of *dementia praecox*, her argument appears circular.

La Démence précoce demonstrates Pascal's early if tentative discussion of psychopathology and psychology, especially the theories of Freud and Jung. She had previously noted the disjunction between gesture and feeling in her patients. She was interested in Carl Jung's early work with seriously demented and catatonic patients, especially his attempts to interpret the significance of the signs and repeated gestures such patients made. Though she qualifies her interest in psychological, as opposed to physiological, aspects of patients' illness somewhat apologetically as a 'digression', her discussion of psychopathology show her eagerness to go beyond a purely nosological model of mental illness and is far more adventurous in this respect than other contemporary accounts of *dementia praecox*.[24]

An important influence on Pascal in this regard was the work of Théodule Ribot (1839–1916), the founder of French psychology in a scientific, as opposed to a purely theoretical sense.[25] As a student in Paris, she may have attended his lectures. Ribot, who had published widely on theories of memory, the will and the emotions, had formulated, well before Freud, the concept of unconscious states in the mind. Automatic behaviour (tics etc.) was for Ribot a manifestation of the unconscious. Below the level of our conscious states, he argued, lies a whole substratum of unconscious memories, sensations, and residues of everyday life. A convinced materialist and positivist, Ribot affirmed that these unconscious phenomena were physiological, not spiritual in origin. In Ribot, Pascal must have seen a way to combine a commitment to the affective reality of her patients' illnesses with her materialist convictions.

Ribot described subconscious influences, independently paralleling Proust's fictional formulations:

> On ne peut nier que les événements quotidiens laissent en nous des impressions fugitives, éphémères, qui ne restent pas dans la conscience et cependant subsistent au-dessous d'elle, excitant à quelque degré des désirs et aversions trop faibles pour se manifester au dehors, mais qui s'organisent par la répétition. Ce sont des petits faits d'expérience gravés dans notre mémoire organique où ils semblent ensevelis pour

24 Barbier, *VOCP*, 83–87.

25 See for example Théodule Ribot, *Problèmes de la psychologie affective* (Paris: Alcan, 1910).

toujours, comme tant d'autres souvenirs que le hasard ressuscite à notre grand étonnement – des impressions éparses de choses vues ou entendues. Ces résidus, similaires ou non, mais qui tous se rapportent à une personne ou à un même objet, agissent dans des conditions favorables; les dispositions deviennent des actes: c'est le soubassement profondément enseveli, ignoré sur lequel la passion naissante trouve un solide point d'appui (*Essai sur les passions*, 18–19).

[One cannot deny that daily events leave fleeting, ephemeral impressions within us, which do not remain in the consciousness and yet survive underneath it, where they go some way to stimulate desires and aversions too weak to be externally perceptible but which form coherent patterns through repetition. They are fragments of actual experience etched into our organic memory where they lie apparently buried, like so many other memories that chance suddenly and astonishingly resuscitates – scattered impressions of things seen or heard. These residues, which may or not be similar but which all relate to a person or to a single object, become active under favourable conditions; tendencies become acts. It is on this deeply buried and forgotten substructure that a new passion rests like a fulcrum.]

Pascal followed Ribot in charting the development of an individual's feelings in relation to others and their progressive dissolution in cases of mental illness. Though Ribot was not a clinician and did not use first-hand experimental data, he linked the normal and the abnormal, the so-called healthy and diseased minds as participating in similar processes. Thus, well before Freud, mental illness was configured not as an exceptional or degenerate state, but as following the same physical laws as those of healthy individuals. What appeared formerly as random acts of madness were part of a pattern where the more recently acquired mental and affective qualities gave way to underlying primary states. Pascal was the first to adopt Ribot's term, 'adhédonie', to indicate the loss of a moral sense, the disinhibitions that mark a stage of mental deterioration.[26] The importance of Ribot's experimental psychology for psychiatrists like Pascal was that he encouraged the study of mental illness in terms of a process of dissolution, following observable laws of association and dissociation.[27]

The concept of 'souvenirs affectifs' [emotional memories] became a key formulation in Pascal's understanding of the psychic processes

26 G. Loas, 'News and Notes', *History of Psychiatry*, 7 (1996), 341–42.

27 A. Binet, 'Ribot et la psychologie scientifique française', *Centenaire de Th. Ribot: jubilé de la psychologie scientifique française 1839—1889—1939* (Agen: Imprimerie Moderne, 1939), 8.

of dissolution. They were validated in her view by the clinical work of Freud and Jung:[28]

> Freud, Abraham et Jung ont démontré par la méthode analytique que les traumatismes psycho-sexuels antérieurs à la puberté laissent des traces profondes dans l'imagination des enfants. Comme chez les hystériques, ces souvenirs sexuels deviennent le point de départ des idées et des hallucinations génitales ('Démence', 179).
>
> [Freud, Abraham and Jung have shown by their analytic method that psycho-sexual traumas arising before puberty leave profound traces in children's imaginations. As with hysterics, these sexual memories become the starting-point of genital ideas and hallucinations.]

Pascal recognized the importance of *souvenirs affectifs* as indicating the way in which all human reality is conditioned by a complex blend of feelings arising out of buried memories. Feelings are thus 'real', in the sense that they construct the world we can know. These early indications of interest in subjectivity would be further elaborated in her later work, especially in *Chagrins d'amour et psychoses* [Sorrows of Love and Psychosis] (1935) and in her interest in the philosopher Henri Bergson. Working in an intellectual climate dominated by positivism and committed to standards of objectivity and a materialist understanding of the mind, Constance Pascal nevertheless began, in *La Démence précoce,* to query the largely nosological approach of her profession, to feel that the classifying of mental illness was not the only key to understanding it. The tension between a scientific point of view and a humane understanding of suffering, already marked in her study of Robert Schumann, was one that would inform Pascal's writing throughout her career. She continued to see her patients as objects for research, indeed to perform experiments on them, but their affective life haunted, mystified and enthralled her.

28 See Ohayon, *L'Impossible Rencontre*, 80–92.

5. Charenton and Prémontré, 1917–22

Pascal returned to Clermont de l'Oise shortly after her daughter's birth on 17 July 1916, but she soon arranged to be seconded in a temporary appointment to the Maison Nationale de Santé at Saint Maurice, a section of the Charenton Asylum on the outskirts of Paris, which had become a military hospital during the war.[1] The Clermont Asylum Director complained to his superiors that her absence left him short-staffed. His concerns emerge in a three-cornered correspondence between himself, Pascal, and the Prefect of the Oise region and in which Pascal demanded her arrears in salary payments. The Director complained repeatedly to the Prefect that he had not had a replacement for Pascal and seems to have made difficulties about payment.[2] They were evidently still on exceedingly bad terms. Writing to the Prefect three years later (24 June 1919), the Director claimed that Pascal had taken leave from Clermont without having first returned to her post, 'Mlle Pascal ayant la fâcheuse habitude d'altérer la vérité' [Mlle Pascal having the regrettable habit of distorting the truth].[3] The Prefect seems to have believed her, as she eventually received her salary. She remained at Saint Maurice until 1920 when she was appointed senior psychiatrist (*médecin-chef*) at the Psychiatric Asylum of Prémontré in the Aisne region in north-eastern France. She was the first woman in France to occupy the post of *médecin-chef.*

Nonetheless, Pascal's transfer from Clermont to what she hoped would be a permanent post at a higher grade proved problematic, partly due to her acrimonious relations with the Director – what a

1 André Rodiet, 'La situation des asiles de la Seine pendant la guerre, et les transferts des aliénés parisiens en province', *Le Progrès médicale* (25 October 1919), 428–29; Gregory Thomas, 'Open psychiatric services in interwar France', *History of Psychiatry*, 15, 2 (2004), 137.

2 18, 22, 29 November 1916, DCPCAC.

3 Constance Pascal, Clermont DACP (1908–21).

civil servant referred to as her 'retentissants démêlés avec l'Asile de Clermont' [resounding disputes with the Asylum at Clermont] and partly to the scarcity of suitable posts as a *médecin-chef*, a promotion which was now overdue.[4] However, her interim period at Saint Maurice was a great liberation after Clermont. She wrote in her Journal:

> Et comme je suis heureuse à Charenton. Quelle vie différente; indépendance dans le travail, calme, respect, dignité; je me retrouve; le service m'appartient. Je fais ce que je veux. L'autre jour j'ai présidé une commission militaire, fait unique dans les annales féministes et c'était très intéressant. J'ai obtenu ce que j'ai voulu avec mes manières simples (CP WJ, April 1917).
>
> [How happy I am at Charenton! What a different life: independence in my work, calm, respect, dignity. I feel myself again. I am in charge of my department, I can do what I want. And the other day I chaired a military commission, a unique event in the annals of feminism, and it was most interesting. I got what I wanted by being simple and straightforward.]

The military authorities, recognizing her competence, had designated her an expert medical witness in cases involving shell-shocked patients. Significantly, Pascal saw her appointment as chair of the tribunal as a feminist victory. Two other phrases in this letter seem characteristic and contrast with her frustrations at Clermont: 'I can do what I want' and 'I got what I wanted by being simple and straightforward'. Somewhat autocratic, though possessed of great charm, Pascal found negotiation, particularly about issues on which she felt strongly in the professional context, difficult and demeaning. This pattern of conflict with the administrations of the asylums where she worked would remain throughout her career.

At Charenton Pascal's domestic life was also eased. She was able to look after her daughter, though she continued to be preoccupied by concerns for her future. Deeply troubled about her daughter's likely fate in the post-war turmoil, fearing that the child would be severely disadvantaged by social stigma because of her illegitimate status, Pascal drafted a will in 1918 leaving her entire estate to Jeanne:

> Et ma Jeannette dans ce pays sans organisation, elle qui a tant besoin de soins, de tant d'amour. Attachée à ma vie, elle subira mon malheureux sort. Mais je crois à mon étoile; depuis qu'elle est là, ma vie est un paradis, et doit durer. J'ai trop souffert dans le passé. Il n'est

4 Note to Conseiller d'Etat de l'Assistance et de l'Hygiène Publiques, DCPCAC (30 April 1920).

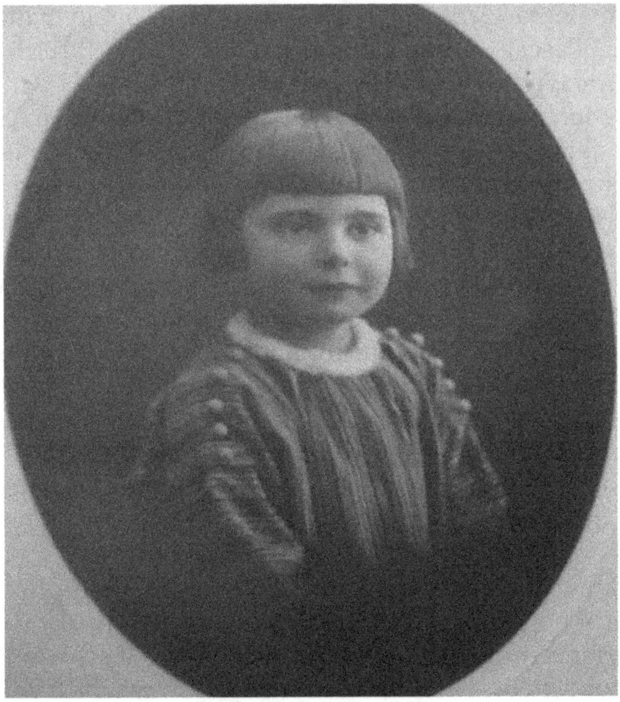

Fig 4. Jeanne Pascal aged three

pas possible que je perde ce bonheur qui me vient si tard. Ma petite Jeanne est une fille qui connaîtra la vie dure; le peu de fortune que je lui laisse lui permettra de supporter plus facilement la vie de misères et de larmes qui l'attend. [...] Je désire que l'éducation de ma petite Jeanne soit faite par mon amie, Mlle Streicher. Que mes amies aient pitié d'elle; c'est un petit être adorable (PRFP, 16 March 1918).

[What will become of my Jeannette in this disordered country – she needs so much to be well cared for and loved! Linked to my life, she will inevitably suffer my unhappy fate. But I believe in my star. Since she has been with me, my life has been a paradise, and this must continue. I have suffered too much in the past. It is simply impossible that I could lose this happiness, which has come to me so late. My little Jeanne is a child who will know hardship. The modest legacy I leave her will allow her to bear more easily the poverty and misfortunes that lie ahead. [...] I wish my little Jeanne's upbringing to be in the charge of my friend Mlle Streicher. May my friends have pity on her; she is an adorable little being.]

A properly notarized will (22 August 1920) again named Jeanne Madeleine Pascal as her sole heir, with Jeanne Streicher as heir, should Jeanne pre-decease her.[5]

Justin Mengin continued to play a key role in the lives of Pascal and their daughter. He lobbied vigorously with the Ministry for her promotions and transfers. Whether, or how long, he and Constance remained lovers is unknown. Jeanne Pascal Rees believed that there were no such relations between her parents in her childhood. The General, known to her as Parrain [Godfather], was a frequent and joyous visitor to their various homes. Thanks to his engineering background, he was a wonderful handyman, his daughter recalled, once building her a radio-set – a technological marvel at the time. He accompanied Constance and Jeanne on many holidays in her childhood.[6] He certainly did not abandon his illegitimate daughter, but nor did he grant her legal recognition. This ambivalence became a source of increasing bitterness to Pascal over the years. To the young Jeanne Pascal, the General was her adored godfather.

At Charenton, having re-established contacts with her friends in Paris, Pascal no longer suffered from the acute sense of isolation she had experienced during the war at Clermont. It was in this period that she published an article on women's suffrage in *La Voix commune* entitled 'La femme française votera-t-elle?'[Will French women vote?] This is her only avowedly feminist piece of journalism, though it is clear from the comment quoted above from her journal that she had strong feminist sympathies. Pascal may have been responding, whether consciously or unconsciously, to a survey held in 1914 by *Le Petit Echo de la Mode* (the women's magazine for which she had written her articles on childcare), to determine whether French women wanted the suffrage. The result, published on 17 May 1914 under the title 'Les femmes veulent-elles voter: oui ou non?' [Do women want the vote or not?] demonstrated that out of an impressive 252,638 women polled, 143,993, or 57%, did not want the vote – though on this occasion they had, ironically, been forced to vote in order to express their desire not to do so. Given the paper's readership the result is not surprising.[7] Pascal's riposte, or intervention in the women's suffrage issue, though delayed by the Great War, suggests that she had shaken off the caution on gender issues of her previous journalistic period:

5 Testament Constance Pascal, 22 August 1920, PRFP.

6 IJPR 15–16 July 2002.

7 Charle, *Le Siècle de la presse*, 193.

> La femme française votera malgré les craintes des sots, les sourires des galantins et la résistance misonéiste de quelques vieillards, parce que le changement de la face du monde exige qu'elle prenne pleinement conscience de ses devoirs de femme, d'épouse et de mère.[8]

> [French women will vote in spite of the fears of fools, the sneers of fops and the misogynistic resistance of a few old men, because the world has changed and this means that they must fully embrace their duties as women, wives and mothers.]

Like many feminists arguing for political suffrage, Pascal underscored the duty of women as citizen-mothers to fulfil what were assumed to be their gender functions in the public as well as in the private sphere. Her scorn for traditionalist male opponents could not be more marked. Her ironic and pugnacious tone suggests both a sense of entitlement and the confidence to speak out on feminist issues.

Pascal devoted much of the year 1919 to bombarding the Ministry with requests for a permanent appointment as *médecin-chef*. Still formally posted to Clermont, though on secondment, she feared that her eleven years there might turn into a permanent exile in a place she hated. An intensely emotional letter to the minister which is preserved in her file, one of the many she wrote at this period, reflects her state of crisis, based on her fear of a return to the isolation of asylum life in the provinces.

> Je ne vous ai pas assez remercié de tout le réconfort moral que vous m'avez donné et de l'intérêt que vous me portez. Si je vous demande un peu de temps pour réfléchir et choisir, c'est que je garde de la province méchante et mesquine les souvenirs les plus douloureux; j'ai encore les nerfs brisés de la lutte que j'ai eue à mener. [...] Le moi est haïssable [Constance is quoting here from Blaise Pascal's *Pensées*], Monsieur, et j'estime que le mien l'est plus que les autres, mais il y a des circonstances qui obligent à parler de soi. Je suis restée <u>huit ans</u> en petite province <u>sans changer</u> et sans être heureuse. Pendant <u>huit ans</u> je n'ai rien eu à demander au Ministère; c'est un bon point. Mais la guerre est venue. J'étais appelée subitement à faire du bien en dehors de ma sphère; j'ai fait plus que mon devoir, et celui des autres [*sic*]. Par reconnaissance, on a abattu sur moi les pires calomnies, les plus infâmes méchancetés. On a conspiré contre moi à la Préfecture, la sous-Préfecture et la Direction à la Préfecture de Beauvais. Il doit y avoir un dossier qui contient les certificats les plus élogieux des seize mois sur ma conduite pendant l'occupation allemande à Clermont. Ci-joints quelques-uns qui me sont restés; ce sont des preuves indéniables de mon dévouement; or, c'est ce dévouement qui m'a changé la vie en

8 Constance Pascal, 'La femme française votera-t-elle?' *La Voix commune* (13 April 1919).

enfer. Un autre à ma place aurait recueilli quelques félicitations de la part de ses chefs. Moi? [*sic*] Il m'a fallu partir.

Si je vous en parle, Monsieur, ce n'est pas pour qu'on manie ce dossier. Je n'ai aucun mérite d'avoir fait les devoirs abandonnés d'un autre. Je vous en parle, pour que vous sachiez qu'un asile de province est un endroit où le cerveau n'a pas d'aliments et où le cœur se brise contre les préjugés, la méchanceté et la bêtise. Voilà pourquoi j'hésite et vous demande à réfléchir. Et puis, je suis vieille et vieillie. J'ai dix ans d'adjuvant dont huit en province. Autrefois, on devenait médecin en chef au bout de 4–5 ans; c'était le bon vieux temps. Avant la guerre, on gravissait l'étape au bout de 8 ans; c'était déjà beaucoup. Mais la guerre a encore allongé l'adjuvat. Ma promotion et celle d'autres attendra 12–14 ans pour l'avancement. C'est trop. Car l'adjuvat est un esclavage non mérité. Ces promotions victimes de la guerre, méritent quelques égards. Je commence mon onzième année de médecin-adjoint! La guerre ne m'a pas rendue riche. Mon traitement n'est pas assez. Bien que célibataire, j'ai de grosses charges. Je ne vois pas la possibilité de faire les frais de ce double déplacement. Pour toutes ces raisons, je demande un répit. Monsieur, excusez-moi d'avoir parlé si longuement de moi. Cela m'a été pénible. Mais cela vous permettra de mieux me comprendre lorsque j'hésite d'accepter une nouvelle place en province.

Dr Pascal (DCPCAC, 15 January 1919).

[I have not thanked you enough for the moral support that you have given me and the interest you have taken in me. If I ask you for a little time to reflect and decide, it is because I have the most painful memories of that backbiting and mean-minded province; my nerves are still shattered by my struggles [...].The self is hateful [Constance is quoting here from Blaise Pascal's *Pensées*], Monsieur, and I am sure mine is more so than others, but under certain circumstances one is forced to speak of oneself. I spent <u>eight years</u> in the provinces <u>without changing</u> and without being happy. For <u>eight years</u> I made no requests to the Ministry; this is a point in my favour. But the war intervened. I was called upon suddenly to do good outside the scope of my normal duties; I did more than my duty, I did that of other people. By way of thanks, the worst slanders were heaped on me, the most shameful malice. Plots were hatched against me at the Prefecture, the Sub-Prefecture and the Beauvais Administration. I am sure there is a file containing the most glowing certificates covering the sixteen months of the German occupation that I spent at Clermont – I enclose a few that are still in my possession; they are the undeniable proofs of my dedication. Yet it was this very dedication that made my life into a hell. Anyone else would have been congratulated by their superiors. I was forced into leaving.

> If I tell you all this, Monsieur, it is not in order to draw attention to my past career; I did nothing particularly meritorious in taking over the duties abandoned by a colleague. I am telling you this so that you can understand that a provincial asylum is a place where one's mind is left without nourishment and one's spirit is broken by prejudice, meanness and stupidity. This is why I hesitate and am asking you to reconsider. Furthermore I am old and growing older. I have been in a junior grade for ten years, eight of them in the provinces. In the past one could expect promotion to *médecin-chef* after four or five years; those were the good old days. Before the war, one moved up after eight years; that was quite a time. But the war has lengthened the period of apprenticeship still further. My contemporaries and I, along with others, are having to wait twelve to fourteen years for promotion. That is too long. Life in the junior grades is an unmerited servitude. The graduates whose career progression has been held back by the war deserve some consideration. I am entering my eleventh year as junior doctor. The war did not make me rich. My salary is insufficient. Although I am single, my expenses are heavy. I do not see how I can afford the costs of this second move. For all these reasons, I am asking for a respite. Monsieur, excuse me for having talked about myself so long. It has been painful for me. But it will allow you to understand better my reasons for holding back from accepting another post in the provinces.
>
> Dr Pascal]

A week later, the Consultative Commission of the Ministry of the Interior rejected Pascal's request for a permanent post at Charenton, on the grounds that it would set the wrong precedent, saying that in any case funds were insufficient for a permanent appointment.[9] Protracted negotiations ensued. In March, still determined to gain a senior post, Pascal was offered an appointment as junior doctor at Saint Maurice-Charenton, which she turned down. In May she again declined a post as junior doctor at Châlons sur Marne.[10] On 26 May she was ordered to Châlons by the Ministry, but pleaded the illness of her brother Trajan, then in Paris, as an excuse. By 17 July 1919, Pascal who had now applied for leave from Charenton too, wrote to the Director that she was leaving the public psychiatric service altogether to set up in private practice.[11]

Whether this last move was bluff, desperation or merely pique, it proved successful. In August 1919 the Ministry offered Pascal the coveted promotion to *médecin-chef* at the Asylum of Pontorson in

9 DCPCAC, 22 January 1919.

10 DCPCAC, 17 May 1919.

11 DCPCAC.

eastern Brittany, which she accepted.[12] But this appointment too hit an unexpected obstacle. The Préfet de La Manche, the *département* where Pontorson is located, wrote to the Minister:

> En réponse à la dépêche du 24 Septembre par laquelle vous avez bien voulu me demander mon avis au sujet de la nomination de Mlle PASCAL comme médecin-chef du quartier d'aliénés de l'hospice de Pontorson, j'ai l'honneur de vous faire connaître qu'aucune femme n'exerçant la médecine dans la Manche, les populations ne sont pas préparées à cette innovation. La Commission administrative de l'hospice elle-même a certaines préventions à cet endroit d'autant plus qu'il s'agit d'un établissement où sont traités des malades des deux sexes. Elle n'accueillerait certainement pas la candidature de Mlle PASCAL (DCPCAC, 9 October 1919).
>
> [In reply to your telegram of 24 September asking my advice on the nomination of Mlle Pascal as *médecin-chef* in the section for the insane at Pontorson Hospital, permit me to inform you that since there are no women doctors practising in the *département* of La Manche the local population is not ready for this innovation. The administrative commission of the hospital has certain prejudices in this regard, all the more as it is an institution where patients of both sexes are treated. The hospital would certainly not welcome Mlle Pascal's candidacy.]

The refusal to accept a woman psychiatrist or indeed any woman doctors in the *département* was not queried by the Minister. Sexual prejudice seemed to be an adequate reason to reject Pascal's candidacy, that neither she nor her supporters queried, which throws further light on the contested entry of women into the professions. For her part she suspected that the Ministry was fabricating excuses for her lack of promotion. A letter from the Director of Social Assistance and Public Hygiene, dated 30 October 1919, that post-dated her final appointment to Prémontré in the Aisne Département as *médecin-chef* on 10 October 1919, indignantly repudiated allegations she had made:

> M. le Préfet de la Manche m'a fait savoir que l'Asile de Pontorson ne donnerait son agrément qu'à la nomination d'un médecin en chef <u>homme</u>. Cette circonstance m'a empêché de poursuivre les négociations que j'avais entamées pour vous faire attribuer ce poste, mais elle m'a également empêché d'en entamer d'autres pour combler cette vacance, car je tiens autant qu'il soit possible à ce que vous soyez nommée et installée avant ceux de vos collègues qui vous suivent sur la liste. C'est vous dire combien est peu fondé le reproche que vous avez formulé '<u>d'avoir casé les promotions entières auprès de</u>

12 DCPCAC, 25 August and 20 September 1919.

vous'. Vous serez, au contraire, nommée médecin en chef avant MM. les Docteurs SIMON, CALMETTES, DUCOSTE et LATREILLE, tous plus anciens que vous et qui ont préféré par raison de convenances personnelles, que leur promotion fût ajournée.Quant à la place de médecin-adjoint à Ville-Evrard, il vous appartient de vous adresser à la Seine pour vous la faire attribuer, mais vous conviendrez avec moi qu'en ce moment où je fais sur votre demande des démarches pour vous faire agréer en qualité de médecin en chef, il ne m'était pas possible d'avancer votre candidature à un poste de médecin-adjoint. (DCPCAC, 30 October 1919)

[The Prefect of the La Manche *department* has informed me that the Asylum of Pontorson will only agree to the nomination of a male *médecin-chef.* This has prevented me from taking further the negotiations that I had begun to have you appointed to this post, but it has also prevented me from starting on any other negotiations to fill the vacancy, because I am determined, if at all possible, to see you appointed and settled ahead of the colleagues who are below you on the list. This should show you how unjustified you are in your accusation that I have slipped in several full applications that were below yours. On the contrary, you will certainly be appointed *médecin en chef* before Drs Simon, Calmettes, Ducoste and Latreille, who are all older than you but who have decided for personal reasons to defer their promotions. As for the post of *médecin-adjoint* at Ville-Evrard, you must apply to the *département* of La Seine for that, but you will agree with me that at the same time that, at your request, I am attempting to gain you the post of *médecin en chef,* it was not possible for me to advocate your appointment for a post of *médecin-adjoint.*]

Prémontré it was to be. Pascal was finally nominated officially to the post on 17 January 1920.[13] She had now gained a key promotion in the psychiatric hierarchy. It was a position of considerable power and responsibility, with administrative as well as medical duties. The *médecin-chef* was responsible for several hundred patients. At Clermont in 1908, for example, there had been only two *médecin-chefs* for 1673 patients, two *médecins-adjoints* – of whom Pascal was one – and four interns. It was the *médecin-chef* who had the power to detain or discharge patients, so the job also incorporated a medico-legal function. Given the numbers of patients involved, the post left little time for purely psycho-therapeutic practice.[14]

It was not the position itself which was daunting. Pascal, now aged 43, was eager to accept professional challenges and to acquire significant responsibility. But to be sent to Prémontré Asylum must

13 17 January 1920, DCPCAC.

14 Barbier,*VOCP,* 18–19.

have been seen within the psychiatric sector as a poisoned chalice. Originally a monastery belonging to the Premonstratensian Order, it became an insane asylum in 1867, retaining a Catholic presence with nuns employed on the nursing staff, although it was a public asylum under the meaning of the 1838 act that had established the state-run asylum system[15]. The seventeenth-and eighteenth-century buildings, in a setting of great natural beauty, lie in a valley surrounded by forests in the mountainous region of Saint Gobain. Because of its geographic position on the Eastern Front, during the 1914–18 war, Prémontré was heavily bombarded from both sides.[16] After the creation of the Hindenberg Line in March 1917, the hospital found itself three kilometres behind enemy lines. Prémontré had the dubious distinction of being the French asylum that had been most heavily damaged in the Great War. Even today one can see in the exterior wall the marks of shell-holes from the pitched battles that took place there.

At the outbreak of war, the director and doctors were drafted to the front and the asylum was left in the charge of the bursar, a M. Letombe, together with his son, who struggled to find food for the 1300 patients in residence in 1914. Some 539 inmates, nearly half the total population, died within the year, of disease, neglect and starvation, a grim precursor to the death toll in psychiatric hospitals under Vichy. The remainder were eventually evacuated to Belgium in 1916 in horrific conditions. The Germans successfully held Prémontré from 1 September 1914 until the end of hostilities. The surviving patients were repatriated only in September 1919. The damage suffered by the buildings was second only to that undergone by the patients. The splendid monastery buildings were left roofless and pitted with shell-holes; all useable equipment was stripped out by the retreating German forces and much of the surrounding forest flattened. When Constance Pascal arrived to take up her post in January 1920, four months after the hospital had reopened, most of the buildings were still in ruins, patients wandered about without food or shelter and Pascal found that the accommodation to which she had been assigned in the hospital grounds was completely uninhabitable. She applied for leave of absence until she and little Jeanne could have a roof over their heads. For the next few months she commuted to Prémontré

15 Goldstein, *Console and Classify*, 301–11.

16 A contemporaneous account of these events is found in Joseph Charpentier, 'Un asile martyr: Prémontré pendant la guerre', *L'Informateur des aliénistes et des neurologistes*, 16e année, 1 (1921), 154–59.

from Saint Maurice, writing icily to the interim director on 26 January 1920:

> J'ai l'honneur de vous faire connaître que j'ai pris possession aujourd'hui de mon poste à l'Asile de Prémontré. Avec l'impossibilité de me loger, j'étais obligée, à mon grand regret, de faire une demande de congé. J'espère, M. le Directeur, que vous [feriez] les réparations urgentes de mon logement afin que je puisse m'installer d'une façon définitive.[17]
>
> [Permit me to inform you that today I have taken up my post at the Asylum of Prémontré. Given the impossibility of residing there, I was forced, to my great regret, to ask for leave of absence. I hope, M. le Directeur, that you will undertake urgent repairs to my lodgings in order that I can take up permanent residence.]

By September, matters had been arranged, as is evidenced by Pascal's request for compensation for rent and removal expenses during her period of commuting from Charenton. However a note to the Minister from a highly irritated civil servant reveals that almost from the moment of her arrival, Pascal had applied not just for a leave of absence but for a permanent transfer from Prémontré:

> Pour répondre à la note par laquelle Monsieur le Conseiller d'État, Directeur de l'Assistance et de l'Hygiène publiques, a demandé si nous disposions en ce moment d'un poste qui pût être attribué à Mlle PASCAL, Médecin en chef de l'Asile public d'aliénés de Prémontré, le Chef du 1er Bureau a l'honneur de lui faire savoir qu'à l'heure actuelle il n'en est aucun de disponible, mais que des vacances se produiront sans doute après le concours de la Seine et qu'il sera possible alors de donner satisfaction à cette doctoresse.
>
> Toutefois il serait peut-être imprudent d'espérer que le cours de ses incessantes réclamations prendrait fin, même dans cette hypothèse: Mlle PASCAL est en effet très difficile à contenter, et ce n'est pas trop m'avancer que de soutenir que, par ses visites, par ses lettres réitérées (quelquefois deux par jour) adressées personnellement au sous-chef de mon bureau, chargé spécialement des affaires concernant les médecins des asiles, par les interventions des personnalités politiques ou médicales en sa faveur, elle donne à mon service plus d'ouvrage à elle seule que la plupart de ses collègues.
>
> Actuellement elle est à Prémontré, au moins nominalement, car en fait elle continue à résider dans le département de la Seine, où elle était, il y a peu de temps, médecin-adjoint en disponibilité à la suite de ses retentissants démêlés avec l'Asile de Clermont. Elle se plaint d'être obligée, dans ces conditions, de s'imposer des frais exorbitants

17 Corr. CP & Director, Prémontré DACP (26 January 1920).

de voyage et de séjour quand elle se rappelle que son devoir exige sa présence à Prémontré. Mais il est bien évident qu'elle pourrait faire évanouir cet inconvénient en occupant son poste, comme le font les autres médecins du cadre. Je conviens que Prémontré, situé en plein pays dévasté, ne peut pas lui offrir tout le confortable qu'elle trouverait dans des asiles appartenant à des régions moins éprouvées, mais elle ne pouvait ignorer, en acceptant ce poste, que les Allemands avaient passé par là et qu'elle ne pouvait, dès lors, compter que sur une installation de fortune. D'autre part, il lui a été répété à satiété, qu'on avait pris bonne note de sa candidature à un autre poste, et cette réponse a été également faite aux nombreux recommandants qu'elle nous a envoyés et qui s'acquittent de leur mission, le plus souvent, en souriant de l'insistance prodigieuse de leur cliente et en s'en excusant auprès de nous (DCPCAC, 30 April 1920).

[In reply to the note in which the *Conseiller d'Etat,* Director of Public Welfare and Hygiene asked if we have currently available a post that could be assigned to Mlle Pascal, *Médecin en chef* at the Public Asylum for the Insane at Prémontré, the Head of the First Section wishes to inform him that at the present time there are no such posts available, but that some vacancies will follow the *concours* [competitive exam] of the Seine *département* and that it should then be possible to satisfy this lady. It would perhaps, nevertheless, be unwise, even in this case, to hope that the incessant flow of her demands might come to an end. Mlle Pascal is in fact very difficult to satisfy and it would not be an exaggeration to say that with her visits, her repeated letters (sometimes two a day) personally addressed to the deputy head of my department, who is in charge of all matters concerning asylum doctors, the representations made by distinguished political or medical persons in her favour, she gives my department more work on her own than most of her colleagues.

At the moment she is at Prémontré, at least in theory, for in fact she continues to reside in the Seine *département,* where she used to be *médecin-adjoint,* on leave following her resounding disputes with the Asylum at Clermont. She complains that this forces her to bear exorbitant travel expenses and the costs of lodging when she remembers that her duties demand her presence at Prémontré. But it is surely obvious that she could do away with this problem by occupying her post, like other doctors at her level. I admit that Prémontré, which is situated in the middle of ravaged lands, cannot offer her all the comforts she might find in less affected asylums, but she must have known when she accepted the post that the Germans had been there and so her lodgings would be makeshift at best. What's more, she has been repeatedly told that her application for another post has been well noted, and this reply has also been given to the many representatives she has sent us and who, most often, carry out their mission with an embarrassed smile, apologizing for the excessive insistence of their client.]

As the above letter indicates, Pascal not only piled on the pressure herself, but enlisted influential friends. Dr Paul Sérieux, General Mengin, the Dean of the Paris Medical School and even the Minister of War all wrote on her behalf. Mengin telephoned the Ministry repeatedly and called in person. A ministerial reply to Paul Sérieux indicates both how much Pascal was respected for her intellect and professional skills and the extent to which her prima-donna-like demands caused annoyance to the Ministry. Pointing out that he could not transfer Pascal until a vacant post became available, the Conseiller d'Etat wrote:

> Autant (et même plus) que Mlle PASCAL, je souhaite qu'elle puisse enfin obtenir un poste que la satisfasse et où elle puisse exercer les qualités d'aliéniste distingué auxquelles vous rendez hommage sans se préoccuper (et sans préoccuper mon administration) de nouvelles demandes de changement. Mais je dois m'en tenir, à son égard comme à l'égard de tous les médecins du cadre, aux principes d'équité qui m'imposent l'obligation de respecter les droits de médecins plus anciens, et quel que soit mon vif désir de la voir pourvue d'un poste à sa convenance, je ne saurais, pour le moment du moins, lui laisser quelque espérance d'obtenir ceux qu'elle sollicite par votre intermédiaire (DCPCAC, 9 July 1920).
>
> [As much as (and even more than) Mlle Pascal, I wish that she may finally find a psychiatric post that satisfies her and where she can exercise those qualities of distinction which you praise, without worrying (or worrying the administration) with repeated requests for transfer. But I have to adhere, in her case as in the case of all doctors of her grade, to principles of fairness which oblige me to respect the rights of longer-serving doctors; and however ardently I might wish to see her provided with a post that meets her requirements, I cannot, for the moment at least, offer her any hope of obtaining those in which she has expressed an interest through your mediation.]

Other posts melted away, either because another candidate had more seniority or because a woman was not thought to carry enough authority or, as in the offer of Agen, because Pascal did not want it.[18] General Mengin lobbied industriously, writing to the Minister:

> Pardonnez-moi de venir vous importuner à nouveau au sujet de la Doctoresse Pascal, et d'appuyer sur les points que je n'ai pu qu'effleurer lors de notre conversation téléphonique. Son plus vif désir, en

18 DCPCAC, 19 July 1920.

quittant Prémontré, serait de pouvoir obtenir le plus tôt possible le poste de Chartres, à défaut de celui de Dun. Je lui ai fait part de vos appréciations très flatteuses au sujet de son service à Prémontré; elle vous en est infiniment reconnaissante, heureuse de mériter l'estime et la bienveillance de ses chefs, par le zèle et la conscience qu'elle apportera toujours dans l'accomplissement de son devoir. De mon côté, je suis particulièrement sensible à l'aimable accueil qui vous voulez bien réserver à mes nombreuses demandes, et vous remercie bien de tout ce que vous pourrez faire pour Mlle Pascal (DCPCAC, 21 July 1920).

[Please forgive me for bothering you once again on the subject of Dr Pascal, in order to stress the points that I could only touch upon in our telephone conversation. Her most ardent wish, on leaving Prémontré, would be to obtain as soon as possible the post at Chartres or, failing that, at Dun [sur-Auron]. I passed on to her your most flattering consideration of her work at Prémontré. She is immensely grateful to you, happy to deserve the esteem and kindness of her directors for the zeal and the commitment with which she will continue to fulfil her duty. For my part, I am particularly sensible of the kind reception you have given to my many requests and I thank you sincerely for all that you can do for Mlle Pascal.]

Alternative posts were suggested, but none of them became available. Sérieux wrote again pleading for the Ministry to put an end to Pascal's exile in the devastated regions.[19] The Dean of the Paris Medical Faculty wrote glowingly:

J'ai l'honneur de vous faire savoir qu'elle a été mon élève; qu'elle a eu une carrière particulièrement brillante et qu'elle a toujours rempli avec autant de science que de dévouement les postes qui lui ont été confiés. Elle a publié un grand nombre de travaux qui lui ont acquis une grande et légitime notoriété (DCPCAC, 30 August 1920).

[Permit me to inform you that she was my student; she has had an exceptionally brilliant career and has always carried out her work in the posts with which she has been entrusted with both scientific skill and dedication. She has a large number of publications, which have justifiably gained her a considerable reputation.]

While this lobbying was in progress, Pascal took up residence at Prémontré in September, eventually receiving compensation for rent and removal expenses during her period of commuting from Charenton. She did not let up her lobbying pressure. By the end of 1920, a civil servant at the ministry sounded thoroughly exasperated:

19 DCPCAC, 21 August 1920.

'Et la Doctoresse Pascal? Je désirais en finir avec ses réclamations incessantes en lui attribuant un poste auquel, étant déjà en fonction, elle peut prétendre par priorité' [As for this Dr Pascal, I was trying to put an end to her incessant demands by finding her an appointment which would be hers by prior claim, since she is already in post] (DCPCAC, 24 December 1920). Her hospital dossier contains no further information until 7 September 1921, by which time she had been in post for a year and a half, when she applied for sick leave. Her ensuing letters to the new, permanent Director, M. Lenoir, reveal that again she had experienced great difficulties and discouragement at Prémontré, just as she had at Clermont – this in spite of cordial feelings towards Lenoir. She clashed with the nursing sisters, finding ingrained resistance to her attempts to reform patient treatment. Although no mention of little Jeanne Pascal, now a lively four-year-old (see letter of 3 September 1920 below), appears in the official record, an inventory of the new doctor's personal effects lists a child's high chair, a reminder that Pascal's move to Prémontré was enriched and complicated by her family situation.

Pascal had three major sources of support in this period. The first, her brother Trajan Pascal, had served in the Romanian Army, was now a colonel and had been appointed as a military attaché to the Paris Peace Conference of 1920–22.[20] Brother and sister had become temporarily reconciled. Trajan's wife Marie and their son Ion (or Jean), about whose care Constance had written at such length to her sister-in-law in 1912, accompanied him to Paris. Constance introduced little Jeanne to her Romanian family as her orphaned foster-child. One legacy of the Great War was that it left some 700,000 French children parentless. Jeanne's status as a war orphan was therefore entirely plausible.[21] Family anecdotes credit Trajan with helping to fund the reconstruction of the beautiful eighteenth-century chapel at Prémontré.[22] Secondly, the Director of Prémontré, M. Lenoir, appointed probably in late 1920 or early 1921, proved to be a sympathetic and enlightened administrator and a good friend. Thirdly, General Mengin, now retired, was much in evidence,

20 See Frank Swain Marston, *The Peace Conference of 1919: Organization and Procedure* (London: Oxford University Press, 1944). For the numbers of delegates and officials sent by each country to the Paris Peace Conference, see Harold William Vazeille Temperley, ed., *A History of the Peace Conference of Paris* (London: Hodder and Stoughton, 1920–24).

21 Ohayon, *L'Impossible Rencontre*, 1–25.

22 IJPR, 15–16 July 2002.

lobbying the Ministry on Pascal's behalf, assisting her in her moves to and from Prémontré and establishing cordial relations with Lenoir.

Installed in her Prémontré home and seemingly reconciled with her brother, Pascal threw herself into the task of rebuilding the asylum and caring for its demoralized and distressed population. Her relationship with Trajan remained uneasy. She harboured intensely competitive feelings towards him that resurfaced in relation to their children's upbringing. The one letter surviving from this period reveals these familial tensions contrasting with the pleasure Pascal took in her daughter:

> Mon cher Trajan,
>
> J'étais étonnée de ne pas recevoir un mot de toi de Roumanie. Je suis parfois meurtrie de ton indifférence. À Charenton tu étais redevenu mon frère; je t'ai perdu ensuite; je ne te retrouve plus. Cela me fait de la peine mais à quoi bon parler ? Je garde la chambre depuis 15 jours; j'ai un commencement de phlébite. Le Ministre de la Guerre qui est un vieil ami à moi, camarade de laboratoire, désire me voir; si je peux j'irai lundi ou mardi à Paris et j'aurai la plus grande joie d'aller chez toi et d'embrasser le petit Jean. Je voulais te demander de me confier Jean; le 16 Septembre je vais avoir une gouvernante anglaise. Mais si tu vas à Lamalou [Lamalou-les Bains, Haut Languedoc], ce sera très bien pour lui. À son retour, je le prendrai avec joie. Ça lui fera plus de bien que de rester enfermé et couvé comme un œuf par ses parents. Et puis il sera obligé de parler français; avec vous il ne fera aucun progrès, surtout que je suis un Maître pion. Tu te rappelles comme je t'ennuyais avec mes corrections; encore un trimestre chez moi et tu possédais la carcasse de la langue. En famille, tu avais un peu perdu. Fais soigner à Lamalou le petit Jean. Fais-le soigner sérieusement. Ton médecin te dira, après un examen du sang, ce qu'il faudra lui faire. Sa maman a l'amour aveugle; elle ne voit pas ce qui choque même les profanes, son teint cadavérique, son esprit terreux; de bons soins et il sera sauvé, crois-moi bien, je n'exagère pas. Le général a une vieille entérite gourmande; il fait des excès. Tous les ans à la même époque, il est malade. Il doit venir me voir demain. Jeannot est une grande fille de campagne, superbe, intelligente. Elle s'est développée socialement dans les bois de Prémontré; elle est allée à l'école et cela lui fait beaucoup de bien. Il faut envoyer Jean à l'école; le contact est une source inépuisable de richesse mentale.
>
> À bientôt, Bons baisers à Jean et bien affectueusement.
>
> C. Pascal (PRFP, 3 September 1920).

> [My dear Trajan,
>
> I was very surprised not to hear a word from you from Romania. Sometimes your indifference hurts me deeply. At Charenton you

were my brother again; then you were lost to me; now I can no longer find you. This saddens me, but what is the use of talking about it? I have been in bed for the past two weeks with the beginnings of phlebitis. The Minister of War, who is an old friend and former laboratory colleague, wants to see me; if I am up to it, I will go to Paris on Monday or Tuesday and I would love to visit you and embrace little Jean. I wanted to ask you to entrust Jean to me; by 16 September I will have an English governess. But if you go to Lamalou [*a spa in the Haut Languedoc*], that will do him a great deal of good. When he is back, I will have him with great pleasure. That will be much better for him than to stay indoors under his parents' over-protective eye. And with me he will have to speak French; with you he won't learn anything more, whereas I know how to stand over him. You won't have forgotten how I used to annoy you with my corrections. But after one more term you had got the basics of the language. Since then, back at home, you have lost quite a bit.

Get little Jean seen at Lamalou. He could do with a proper check-up. Your doctor should give him a blood test and then tell you what treatment he needs. His mama is blinded by her love for him; she does not see what is obvious even to the layman – his shocking pallor, his sullen state of mind. With proper care he will be saved; believe me, I am not exaggerating.

The General has his usual enteritis, brought on by over-indulgence. Every year at the same time he falls ill. He is coming to see me tomorrow.

Jeannot [*her daughter Jeanne*] is a strapping country girl now, beautiful and intelligent. She is developing socially in the countryside around Prémontré; she has started school and this is doing her a lot of good. You should send Jean to school; it is an inexhaustible source of intellectual enrichment.

See you soon, kisses to Jean, affectionately, C. Pascal]

In addressing her brother, Pascal shifts and weaves through a variety of strategies. From the initial reproaches for neglect, followed by a description of being so ill that she is housebound, Pascal announces a trip to Paris to see her influential friend – probably André Lefèvre (Minister of War from 20 January 1920 to 16 December), who had written in her support to the Ministry of Health.[23] Her offer to take on the care of Trajan's son, Ion, for the duration of what appears to be an extended stay in France, might not have appealed to his parents as it implied criticism of their parenting methods, and the cosseted life that his aunt thinks has made him ill. Marie Pascal, his mother,

23 Jean Jolly, *Dictionnaire des parlementaires français de 1888–1940* (Paris: Presses Universitaires de France, 1966–77).

figures in Pascal's account as a too doting mother, yet if we recall Pascal's pre-war letters to her sister-in-law, she had urged precisely such suffocating care.[24]

In contrast to Ion's [Jean's] allegedly gloomy and unhealthy mien, Pascal writes with genuine pleasure about her daughter. Giving her the nickname Jeannot, usually reserved for boys – 'Johnny' – she suggests a healthy tomboy, which by implication contrasts with the fragile, even feminized, Ion. It appears as a strikingly degendering move.[25] Jeannot figures as a child of nature, unlike her sickly cousin, given the freedom to play in the woods and to attend a local school (though to be supplemented by an English nanny). Pascal's expressed pleasure in her lovely child is moving, if slightly tarnished by the sense that she was engaged in a competition with her brother to establish the excellence of Jeannot's upbringing and more profoundly to contrast her own child, who she cannot acknowledge as hers, as superior to Trajan's son.

The other intriguing detail to emerge concerns Pascal's ironic reference to General Mengin's gastric complaint, demonstrating that he was a member of Pascal's circle and acquainted with Trajan and his wife, though they did not know that he was Jeanne's father any more than they knew she was Jeanne's mother. By 1920, Pascal had established an emotional distance between herself and Mengin. He remained a key part of her life until his death, admiring of her achievements, loyal and supportive and protector of their child, but possibly due to his increasing age, no longer her lover. Nevertheless, the energy and optimism that Pascal expresses in this letter soon failed her. One year later in writing to M. Lenoir, she seems on the point of mental and physical collapse. What in addition to its material challenges were the pressures that made her post at Prémontré intolerable?

Whereas at Clermont de l'Oise Pascal had chafed under the dictatorial sway, as she saw it, of the petty-minded director, at Prémontré her principal difficulties arose with nuns on the nursing staff, who apparently resisted her attempts to reform punitive practices against asylum patients and whom she accused of living in the Dark Ages:

> J'ai senti de loin plus que de près, le bouleversement que j'ai produit dans ces Êtres qui datent de Mérovée et de Pépin-le-Court. J'ai

24 Corr CP & MP, PRFP (2 September 1912) – and see pp. XX of this volume.

25 I am grateful to Naomi Segal for drawing this point to my attention.

> renversé: idées, croyances et habitudes! Dans ce milieu encaissé, l'air nouveau d'une civilisation vivante ne pourra pénétrer qu'avec peine.[26]
>
> [Since I have been away, more than when I was living there, I have come to understand what an upheaval I brought to those Beings who still live in the medieval dark ages of Pépin le Court. I overturned everything: their ideas, beliefs and customs. Nothing is harder than to bring the fresh air of contemporary civilization into that closed world.]

Pascal's problems at Prémontré reflected in part the struggle between clerical and anti-clerical forces in psychiatry that stretched from 1838 to the *Belle Époque*, with both sides seeking to retain control of the psychiatric sector.[27] For psychiatrists, a clerical presence in mental hospitals implied a pre-or anti-scientific approach to treating the mentally ill. For example, in a report on the asylums of western France published in 1901, Dr A. Marie accused the nuns in charge of lacking any understanding of the principles of mental medicine.[28] The psychiatric profession defined the problem as a conflict between science and religious obscurantism. Though this struggle between clerical and lay powers played itself out on the political stage, as well as in the efforts of the psychiatric profession to establish its institutional legitimacy, Pascal's experience demonstrates that on the ground, where religious orders held sway over the nursing staff, psychiatrists who were dependent on the nursing nuns for the patients' day-to-day care could find their ambitions for reform blocked. Pascal's difficulties rested partly on the fact that authority over the nursing sisters was vested in their mother superior, not in the clinical medical staff, as it would have been in a lay institution. The despair and frustration expressed in her letters to M. Lenoir demonstrate to what extent she had reached an impasse at Prémontré.

In other hospitals where she worked, Pascal enjoyed excellent relations with the nursing staff, but it is also the case that given her desire for change and her impatience with those who opposed her, difficulties were bound to arise. For her patients Pascal had inexhaustible sources of compassion; but she was intolerant of opposition. Further, as a single woman and the only woman psychiatrist, she must have seemed a threatening figure to the

26 Corr CP & M Lenoir, Prémontré DACP (3 October 1921). Pascal probably meant Pépin le Bref, b. 714, father of Charlemagne, here a short-hand for the allegedly unenlightened thinking of the dark ages.

27 Goldstein, *Console and Classify*, 361–77; Dowbiggin, *Inheriting Madness*, 1–10.

28 *La Fronde*, BMD (20 January 1901).

traditionalists on the staff, male and female. Pascal was aware that her sex told against her at Prémontré. She felt distrusted and disparaged, resenting the lack of liberty, which Édouard Toulouse had noted, constraining unmarried women.[29] She felt herself the subject of gossip, referring to: 'ces dames de Prémontré qui se sont toutes occupées de mon insignifiante personne' [the ladies of Prémontré who spent all their time discussing my insignificant self].[30] Were inferences drawn, as seems quite possible, about the true parentage of little Jeanne? In September 1921, she wrote to Lenoir, expressing considerable bitterness:

> Pour vous aussi, mon départ sera nécessaire. On n'osera plus dire, lorsqu'un jeune confrère à barbe et à moustaches sera votre très distingué collaborateur, que vous êtes là pour étayer une incapacité.[31]
>
> [For you too, it is high time I left. When your distinguished collaborator is a young person with a beard and moustaches no one will dare to say you only exist to prop up a useless colleague.]

In the course of Pascal's residence at Prémontré, M. Lenoir submitted two annual reports (*apréciations personnelles*) for her dossier, passed on to the Prefect and then the Ministry. They highlight her strengths as a clinical psychiatrist and her weaknesses with regard to her colleagues. The first was entirely positive:

> Mlle le Docteur Pascal a fait preuve depuis son arrivé à l'asile de Prémontré du plus grand dévouement en assumant seule le traitement de près de 300 malades. Très active, Mlle Pascal rend de signales services à l'administration (DCPCAC, 11 February 1921).
>
> [Since she arrived at Prémontré, Dr Pascal has demonstrated the greatest dedication, taking on single-handed the care of some three hundred patients. She is extremely energetic and gives excellent service to the organization.]

The second report was more nuanced, pointing to personality conflicts as well as praising Pascal's professional competence and energy:

> Le Docteur Pascal s'est fait remarquer par son zèle agissant et par son dévouement extrême durant toute la période où elle a exercé à Prémontré. D'un caractère parfois difficile, elle témoigne trop souvent dans ses jugements et ses attitudes d'une partialité qui lui aliène à la longue les bonnes volontés les meilleurs mais son attachement à

29 Huteau, *Psychologie*, 241.

30 Corr CP & Lenoir, Prémontré DACP (9 September 1921).

31 Corr CP & Lenoir, Prémontré DACP (25 September 1921).

ses malades et sa haute conscience ne sauraient être mis en doute (DCPCAC, 6 February 1922).

[The energy, zeal and extreme commitment of Dr Pascal have been striking throughout the time she has been at Prémontré. Having a somewhat difficult personality, her decisions and attitudes too often demonstrate a bias which may in the long run alienate even those best disposed towards her, yet her dedication to her patients and her entire conscientiousness cannot be doubted.]

Whether or not a male psychiatrist with strong views on the care of his patients would have been described as 'having a somewhat difficult personality', the fact is that even the well-disposed M. Lenoir felt constrained to note Pascal's poor relations with some staff.

For her part, Pascal's letters to Lenoir during her extended period of leave from September 1921 until January 1922, convalescing from a combination of rheumatism and depression, express her sense of defeat as well as her gratitude for his many kindnesses:

Je me repose mal à cause des soucis constants et de la fatigue morale que je sens d'avantage aujourd'hui. Il était temps que je parte. [...] Permettez-moi de vous remercier de toutes vos exquises délicatesses. Le général m'a chargé de vous transmettre avec ses bons souvenirs ses sentiments de reconnaissance pour tout ce que vous avez fait pour lui à Prémontré.[32]

[I am not finding it easy to rest because I am increasingly plagued by the constant worry and emotional exhaustion. It was certainly high time I left. [...] But let me thank you for all your exquisite tact and kindness. The General wishes to be remembered to you and has also asked me to pass on his gratitude for everything you did for him at Prémontré.]

Now retired from the army, the General was a regular visitor. It is possible that the Director may have been privy to Pascal and Mengin's domestic situation.

While on leave, Pascal hoped to apply for grade of *médecin-chef* in the Seine region, which had a separate *concours*. It was the last hurdle she had to overcome in the psychiatric hierarchy and her chance to return permanently to Paris.[33] She was not alone among psychiatrists in seeing this as the ultimate prize. The competition was intense, but the examination that year was postponed – due to lack of vacant posts or, as Pascal commented acidly:

32 Corr CP & Lenoir, Prémontré, DACP (9 September 1921).

33 Barbier,*VOCP*, 19–21.

Les vieillards de Ste Anne, fortement soutenus, ne veulent pas partir à 70 ans! Ils m'ont obstrué la circulation. Donc concours remis aux calendes grecques. En province, la circulation est barrée aussi par les séniles, hors d'usage. Les lois sont faites pour les professeurs, pas pour tous.[34]

[The old men of Ste Anne are sitting pretty; they are not ready to retire at seventy! They are blocking my promotion. So the *concours* is postponed till the end of time. It's the same in the provinces: all movement is blocked by those senile old duffers. It's one law for the professors, another for the rest of us.]

A sense of failure and frustration dominate her letters to Lenoir. Referring to an article she had recently published, she told him: 'En le lisant, vous sentirez combien j'aime mes malades. Leur bien-être et mon métier, c'est toute ma vie. C'est pourquoi j'ai beaucoup souffert de n'avoir pas pu le faire comme je le voulais' [When you read it you will understand how much I love my patients. Their well-being and my profession is my whole life. That's why it was so painful for me not to be able to do what I wished].[35]

Pascal's professional interests overlap in these letters with her personal concerns. Her remarks about a patient at Prémontré, a M. Navarre, could have applied to herself and General Mengin. Navarre's wife was seeking a divorce on the basis that her husband was incurably insane and possibly syphilitic. As noted previously, the law of 1884, liberalizing divorce in France, forbade it in cases of patients interned in asylums.[36] Pascal had applied the Wasserman Test for syphilis to Navarre and, if positive, this would have given his wife grounds for divorce. However, the test proved negative. Faced with this intractable situation, Pascal comments:

Il y a à la bibliothèque un livre sur le divorce des aliénés: sur la première page: une femme enchaînée à un fou! C'est M. Navarre. Mais que peut-on faire contre la loi ? J'ai vu défiler dans mon bureau beaucoup de maris qui veulent couper la laisse; rien à faire.[37]

[In the library there is a book on the divorce of the insane. The very first page features the case of a woman shackled to a madman! It is

34 Corr CP & Lenoir, Prémontré, DACP (25 September 1921).

35 Corr CP & Lenoir, Prémontré, DACP (25 September 1921), Constance Pascal, 'La Suppression des garderies de fous', *La Presse Médicale* (September, 1921), 1389–91.

36 Murat, 2001, 290–92.

37 Corr CP & Lenoir, Prémontré DACP (25 September 1921); Copy of the Rules and the Jury for the *Concours de médecin chef des asiles de la Seine* (DCPCAC).

M. Navarre to the life. But what can one do against the law? Plenty of husbands have trooped through my office wanting to cut the leash; there is nothing I can do.]

General Mengin may well have been one of those husbands, who initially came to Pascal for advice on cutting the leash.

While on leave at Saint Maurice, Pascal assisted her former mentor at Ville Evrard, Dr Paul Sérieux, with reconstruction plans for the Maison Blanche Asylum. The post-war period provided unrivalled opportunities for the reconstruction of neglected or ruined buildings. Dr Sérieux was engaged in supervising new building projects based on his model pavilions at Ville Evrard. These plans for physical improvements led Pascal on to discuss medical improvements, which of course had financial implications. Writing to Lenoir, Pascal argued for investment in the early detection and treatment of syphilis. The victims of this scourge, traditionally and erroneously classified as suffering from general paralysis, an incurable degenerative condition as it was thought, swelled the numbers of patients in French asylums. The funds needed for early diagnosis, she believed, were justified on both humanitarian and economic grounds. Comparing the relative wealth of Parisian asylums and the provinces she remarked:

> Évidemment sans argent on ne pourra rien faire, mais il faut penser à l'économie de l'avenir. Guérir un fou, ce n'est pas seulement mettre sur pied un homme, mais encore alléger le budget d'un pays. Je pense souvent à tous ces syphilitiques non traités qui ont fait souche et qui encombrent les asiles. Traités à temps, quelle économie. C'est là, l'idée du service ouvert; traités à temps, non avec l'oblate mais avec un traitement rationnel.[38]
>
> [Obviously this requires funding, but one must think of longer-term economies. Curing someone of madness is not simply a way of putting a person back on his feet, it also makes savings in the national budget. I often think of all those untreated syphilitics who have taken root and fill up the asylums. Had they been treated in time, what a saving could have been made. That's the whole idea of open surgeries; such patients would be treated before it gets too late, not with oblations but with a rational cure.]

By the end of 1921, Pascal had succeeded in effecting a transfer to the Asile Public d'Aliénés [Public Insane Asylum] at Châlons sur Marne. She received her official appointment as *médecin-chef* on 25

38 Corr CP & Lenoir, Prémontré DACP (25 September 1921). For the development of *service ouvert* see Gregory M. Thomas, 'Open psychiatric services in interwar France', *History of Psychiatry*, 15 (2) (2004), 131–53.

January 1922, taking up her post on 7 February.[39] General Mengin oversaw her removal, writing to M. Lenoir on 14 February:

> Je rentre de Châlons où je viens d'accompagner le Docteur Pascal, et j'ai eu la satisfaction de voir qu'elle allait profiter d'une installation où rien n'a été ménagé au point de vue confort. Les temps sont changés et je revois par la pensée l'arrivée à Prémontré. Je ne veux faire aucune comparaison, mais je me plais à reconnaître les efforts constants que vous avez faits pour améliorer la situation, et je ne doute pas que si vous recevrez les crédits nécessaires, vous n'arriviez à rendre le poste sinon enviable, du moins très supportable pour le successeur du Docteur. Je compte aller vous voir vers la fin mars pour terminer le déménagement, et je vous serais très reconnaissant de vouloir bien faire préparer un cageot pour les poules et un petit cadre pour la glace de l'armoire.
>
> Mengin[40]
>
> [I have just returned from Châlons where I accompanied Dr Pascal and had the satisfaction of seeing that she will have the benefit of accommodation in which no attention has been spared to ensure her comfort. Times have changed – I recall our arrival at Prémontré. I do not mean to make any invidious comparisons; I am most appreciative of the constant efforts you made to improve the situation, and I am quite sure that if you had the necessary funding, you would succeed in making the post if not enviable, at least quite bearable for the Doctor's successor. I will come and see you towards the end of March to complete the removals and would be most grateful if you would get ready a cage for the chickens and packaging for the wardrobe mirror.
>
> Mengin]

The General's reference to poultry highlights another aspect of a psychiatrist's daily existence. Living on the asylum grounds, as they were forced to do, staff benefited from some rural advantages: vegetables from the asylum farm, rabbits and chickens kept for the table and no doubt pork from the piggery. Mengin appeared to enjoy dealing with Pascal's domestic arrangements.

When considering Pascal's time at Prémontré, and her correspondence with M. Lenoir, we are reminded of her pre-war letters to Trajan, detailing manifold complaints about her health, both physical and mental. An example from her farewell letter to the Director can be taken as characteristic:

39 Préfet du Département de l'Aisne to Directeur des Services Administratifs Prémontré, Prémontré DACP and DCPCAC (3 February 1922).

40 Corr Justin Mengin & Lenoir, Prémontré DACP (14 February 1922).

J'ai quitté le lit hier et je me traîne, en boitant dans la maison. Je suis surtout épuisée moralement, fatiguée intellectuellement. Sensible, j'ai souffert de tous les affronts, de toutes les calomnies, en silence: j'ai eu tort, mais on ne peut se refaire. Quel dommage que vous n'ayez pas été dès le début à l'asile; je n'aurais pas tant souffert. J'ai d'autant plus souffert que partout ailleurs j'étais estimée, appréciée: j'ai eu la sympathie de tout le monde. Il m'a fallu venir à Prémontré pour connaître des gens misérables. Ce souvenir ne s'efface pas.[41]

[I got up from my sickbed yesterday and now I'm dragging myself about, limping through the house. Above all, I'm exhausted spiritually, my mind is worn out. I'm too sensitive: I put up with all those insults and slanders in silence. I was wrong, but that's the way I am. What a pity that you were not at the asylum from the beginning; I would not have suffered so much. It was all the more painful for me because everywhere else I have been valued and appreciated. Everyone was my friend. The first time I ever came across such petty, miserable people was at Prémontré. I shall never forget it.]

When Pascal writes that her short tenure at Prémontré represented her first experience of rejection and of meeting 'petty, miserable people', she seems to have forgotten her almost identical reaction to the Clermont administration. Her energy and enthusiasm alternating with despair, and her disdain for her critics remained an emotional pattern throughout her career. Pascal's official profile too reflected these facets of her character. It was recognized that she was legitimately ambitious to rise in the medical-psychiatric hierarchy, devoted to her work and to her patients, but that she consistently antagonized asylum administrators. She could be autocratic and inflexible and was prone to emotional outbursts. On the other hand her supporters, men of distinction in the profession and in public life, admired her brilliance and professional commitment.

Although Pascal had achieved so much professionally, her letters convey a sense that she could not meet her own high standards and that she never felt sufficiently valued by others. They also reflect the pressures of institutional existence on a professional woman, who led a complex private life as a single mother. As in her letters to Trajan where she strove to overturn her subordinate position as a daughter in the traditional Romanian male-oriented household of her childhood, she may have feared that she was in danger of re-experiencing the same subordination in a largely male profession. Pascal's fraught relations with her brother, whom she described as a

41 Corr CP & Lenoir, Prémontré DACP (1 October 1921).

bullying monster but whom she also loved, seem to underpin much of her subsequent mental distress.[42]

The expressions of personal misery, dejection and self-doubt that occur frequently in Pascal's correspondence and in the official files seem the more surprising because they convey the very opposite of her public image. A completely different perspective on her Prémontré sojourn emerges in an article in *La Française* of 1925. The journalist, Élise Émile-Magne, lauding this first woman psychiatrist in the Seine region, described Pascal's experiences, one may feel legitimately, as a heroic enterprise. Here was none of the doubt and discouragement of her letters but an inspirational account of continuous achievement. Apart from Pascal herself, Magne may have interviewed some of her friends. In this account, the Prémontré episode takes its place in a narrative of feminist progress:

> En 1920, il faut pourvoir d'un médecin-chef l'asile de Prémontré. Cet asile a été dévasté et en partie détruit par la guerre; tous les confrères en refusent la charge; Mlle Pascal, vaillamment, l'accepte. Et ceux qui s'en vont visiter les ruines de cette merveilleuse abbaye de Prémontré, si ravagée par les obus, s'étonnent de trouver là cette jeune femme, installée dans un logis sans toit et sans fenêtres, presque à la merci de ses aliénés, pour lesquels elle ne dispose même point d'une cellule, en cas d'accès furieux. Mais qu'importe? 'Ce n'est pas cela qui me manque le plus, dit-elle à ses amis inquiets; ce sont les baignoires, les réfectoires, les infirmières, une pharmacie. Et, malgré les difficultés accumulées, deux ans suffisent à son énergie pour combler les lacunes qui la désolent; les chiffres à ce sujet sont probants: avant l'arrivée de Mlle le Docteur Pascal à Prémontré, on enregistrait douze à quinze décès par jour; quand elle quitta cet asile en 1922, on n'en avait pas constaté un seul depuis cinq mois.[43]

> [In 1920, a consultant doctor was needed for the asylum of Prémontré. This asylum was laid waste; it had been partly destroyed in the war; all the eligible practitioners refused the post. Mlle Pascal courageously accepted it. And those who paid a visit to the ruins of this wonderful Prémontré abbey, so ravaged by shells, were amazed to find this young woman, living in accommodation without a roof or windows, almost at the mercy of her mad patients, for whom she did not even have one secure cell in case of a violent outbreak. But what did that matter? 'That is not what I most need,' she said to her concerned friends; 'what we are short of are baths, dining rooms, nurses and a pharmacy'. And yet, in spite of all these problems, it took just two

42 IJPR 17 June 2003.

43 Élise Émile-Magne, 'La première femme aliéniste de la Seine', *La Française* (PRFP, 1925).

> years for this energetic woman to make good those gaps she found so worrying. The statistics are conclusive: before Mlle Pascal's arrival at Prémontré, twelve to fifteen deaths were recorded every day; when she left in 1922, there had not been a single death for five months.]

Though it seems to contradict in almost every detail Pascal's hesitations in undertaking the Prémontré post and her misery-laden letters to M. Lenoir, Émile Magne's article can be seen nevertheless as representing a true though partial aspect of Pascal's persona. Throughout her career, especially within the hospital setting, as is clear from numerous press reports, she gave an impression of poise, authority and charm. However, given the isolation of asylum life, where senior staff were few and social relations with colleagues limited, where staff were obliged to live 'on campus' and therefore not in a town or village setting and, given that a single woman in this setting would experience intense surveillance of her private life, it is scarcely surprising that Dr Constance Pascal, intelligent, highly strung and ambitious, should have expressed her loneliness and fits of personal despair to those few individuals with whom she was able to be intimate or who she felt were her allies. At the same time, her relentless lobbying of the Ministry reflects her determination to use every means at her disposal both to advance her career and to ensure a secure life for her daughter.

6. Châlons sur Marne, 1922–25

Pascal's appointment to the Asylum of Châlons sur Marne (now Châlons en Champagne), as *médecin chef des services des femmes* [consultant for women's services] on 25 January 1922, brought freedom from the tensions of Prémontré and welcome new opportunities. Her

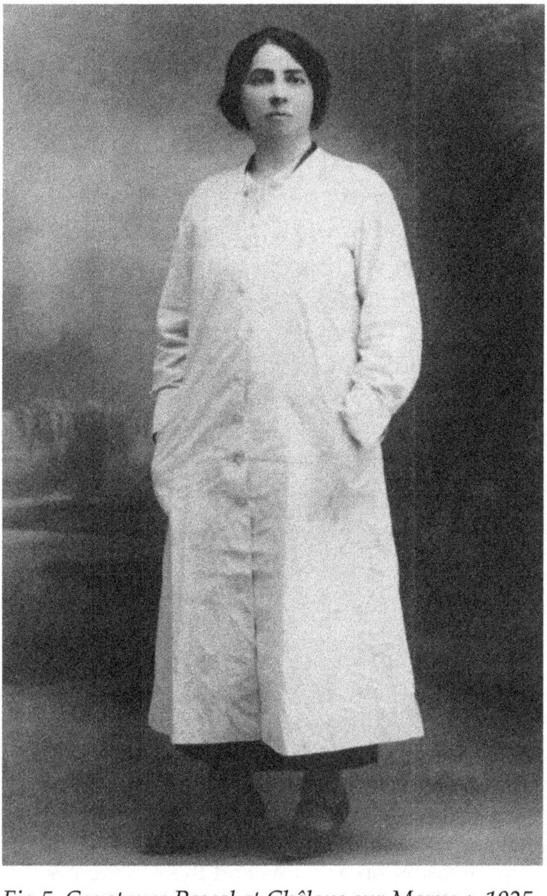

Fig 5. Constance Pascal at Châlons sur Marne c. 1925

salary rose to 12,000 francs. She was made temporary Director pending the appointment of a permanent head.[1] She and her daughter were assigned a comfortable house on the outskirts of the hospital, a great improvement on her Prémontré accommodation, as General Mengin had noted (Prémontré DACP, 14 February 1922). Immediately after taking up her duties, Pascal turned her attention to the creation of open services for children with learning difficulties (the so-called '*handicappés*' or '*anormaux*'), a project, which she had long cherished and which she was the first in France to implement.

Châlons lay in the heart of the Marne region. When Pascal arrived there it was traumatized, like the rest of France, in the aftermath of its demographic catastrophe, the loss of a whole generation of young men.[2] The war had devastated large areas of the countryside, ruined champagne production and dispossessed the agricultural workforce.[3] The hostilities, which had fallen particularly heavily in the Marne region, had disrupted asylum provision, here as elsewhere in France, a situation already familiar to Pascal at Prémontré. Between 1914 and 1918, over 20,000 patients in Parisian asylums were evacuated to the provinces, with the result that provincial asylums became even more overcrowded than formerly.[4] However, after the armistice, many were repatriated, with the result that psychiatric hospitals like Châlons had spare capacity, perhaps for the first time. Pascal moved rapidly and with considerable diplomatic finesse to take advantage of this situation for the creation of her school-clinic for children with severe learning difficulties.

She began with a scheme that must have endeared her to the asylum's Commission de Surveillance [Board of Supervisors] by proposing to save them money. At a meeting of the Commission on 15 April 1922, Pascal presented her objection to plans drawn up by the *département*'s Architect, M. Gélin, to rebuild parts of the hospital and to remodel her own quarters. Gélin's plans entailed an expenditure of 80,000 francs for two new day rooms for paying patients, and

1 Ministry of the Interior, DCPCAC, 25 January 1922.

2 Ohayon, *IR*, 14–21.

3 Hugh Donald Clout, 'Rural revival in Marne, 1914–1930', *Agricultural History Review*, 42: II (1993), 140–55.

4 André Rochet, 'La situation des asiles de la Seine pendant la guerre et les transferts des aliénés parisiens en province' [The situation of insane asylums in the Seine region during the war and the transfer of Parisian mental patients to the provinces] *Le Progrès médical* (25 Octobre, 1919), 428–29. For an analysis of the ever-growing pressure on asylums and their overcrowding in the inter-war period, see Bueltzingsloeven, *HF*, 248–64.

expensive cork flooring in Pascal's house. She convinced the Board of Supervisors that Châlons now had so few paying patients that the new expense could not be justified and suggested that in her own house, central heating would be both more economical and warmer than the proposed flooring. Overall, she proposed improvements that would save the Commission 45,000 francs, a plan that was unanimously adopted.[5]

With this leverage, and spare capacity for a time at the asylum, Pascal lodged a formal proposal with the Commission (21 June 1922) for the creation of a special department for mentally and physically handicapped children [*service spécial pour enfants anormaux*]. She was initially opposed by the newly appointed Director who was not yet in post. Alarmed by the fall in the patient population after the war (reduced to half the usual number), he proposed taking patients from over-crowded asylums in the Seine Region.[6] His suggestion was rejected by the Commission, who instead endorsed Mlle Pascal's proposal to use the extra space currently available to found a specialist service for 'les enfants des deux sexes, anormaux et aliénés' [abnormal and insane children of both sexes] from the Marne region. Pascal informed the Commission that having had the opportunity to care for many children suffering from mental disturbances, she was conscious of the great advantages in treating them in their home areas. At present, such children were placed in hospitals outside their own regions, far from their families, which was a source of frequent complaints by parents. The Commission accordingly assigned two currently empty wings of the hospital to Pascal for her new clinic, adding that extensive provisioning and remodelling for the new inmates would be necessary and approving an expenditure of 22,000 francs.[7] On 9 October 1922, Pascal received the Prefect's formal authorization:

> Mlle PASCAL, docteur en médicine, médecin-chef à l'asile d'aliénés, est nommée, avec effet du 1er Octobre 1922, Directrice du Service spécial pour les enfants des deux sexes, anormaux ou aliénés, en

5 Extrait du registre des délibérations de la Commission de Surveillance, Asile Départemental d'Aliénés de Châlons-sur-Marne, Châlons DACP, AM (15 April 1922).

6 Rapport de la Commission de Surveillance, Châlons DACP, AM (21 June 1922).

7 Rapport de la Commission de Surveillance, Châlons DACP, AM (21 June 1922).

> voie d'organisation dans cet établissement; il lui sera adjoint, pour l'enseignement, une Institutrice publique laïque.[8]
>
> [Mlle Pascal, who is a medical doctor and the consultant at the insane asylum, has been appointed with effect from 1 October 1922 as Director of the Special Service for abnormal or insane children of both sexes, which is being set up in this establishment. Primary-level teaching will be provided by a state-trained [non-religious] female teacher.]

Pascal's initiative in the care and education of children with acute special needs formed part of a larger debate in French psychiatry concerning the desirability of instituting 'services ouverts' and the diagnosis, treatment and education of children with learning difficulties.[9] It tied in with the Third Republic's projects to reform public welfare, beginning with the Law of 12 December 1892, amended and strengthened in 1893 and 1905, which provided that 'every Frenchman deprived of financial resources shall receive without charge [...] medical aid in the home, or, if he cannot be effectively cared for there, in an *établissement hospitalier*' [hospital setting].[10] The cost to *départements* of caring for the poor and infirm was partially covered by central government. This helps to explain the enthusiasm of the Châlons Commissioners for Pascal's new children's services, which would fall, as noted by Brisac, the Prefect of the Marne, under the law of 15 July 1893 on medical assistance and the law of 14 July 1905 on the infirm and incurable.[11] A long-time champion of social reform and welfare provision, who had been active in rebuilding the war-ravaged Marne region, Brisac wrote to Paul Strauss, *Ministre de Hygiène, de l'Assistance et des Prévoyances Sociales* [Minster of Public Health, Welfare and Social Planning], outlining Pascal's plan. His letter breathes the contemporary spirit of enlightened republicanism, setting out the humane case for the education and care of children with mental or physical impairments, in the context of the movement for 'open services':

8 Asile Départemental d'Aliénés de Châlons-sur-Marne.

9 Claude Rollet-Echalier, *La Politique à l'égard de la petite enfance sous la Troisième République* (Paris: Presses Universitaires Françaises, 1990).

10 Chambre des Députés, *Débats* (12 December 1892), 654, quoted in John H. Weiss, 'Origins of the French welfare state: poor relief in the Third Republic, 1871–1914', *French Historical Studies* XIII: 1 (1983), 47–77.

11 Corr Prefect & the Director, Asile Départemental d'Aliénés de Châlons-sur-Marne, Châlons DACP, AM (9 October 1922).

J'ai l'honneur de vous rendre compte que j'ai décidé de créer dans le Département de la Marne, un service spécial pour les enfants anormaux et que, par délibération du 12 Septembre 1922, le Conseil Général a approuvé mon projet et voté les crédits nécessaires à sa réalisation. À l'heure actuelle, en effet, il n'existe dans le Département aucun établissement destiné à recevoir les enfants anormaux, à les soigner et à les éduquer; les petits invalides cérébraux doivent être envoyés dans d'autres départements afin de suivre le traitement médico-pédagogique nécessaire à leur développement. [...]

Le Service nouveau, véritable Institut médico-pédagogique recevra les catégories suivantes d'enfants anormaux, âgés de moins de 16 ans.

1. les enfants des deux sexes, curables ou perfectibles et socialement adaptables, appelés, par conséquent, à bénéficier des dispositions de la loi d'instruction du 15 avril 1909.
2. les enfants des 2 sexes inéducables et socialement inadaptables, le poids mort de la société, les épileptiques-psychopathes, les imbéciles, les idiots, les infirmes cérébre-médullaires à qui des soins sont constamment nécessaires.

Vous estimerez sans doute avec moi, Monsieur le Ministre, que ces enfants qui ne constituent pas un danger pour la sécurité publique, ne doivent pas être placés sous le régime de la loi de 1838, et que, par suite, ce service spécial doit être un service ouvert. [...] En l'état actuel de l'Assistance des anormaux, tout enfant arriéré est stigmatisé de l'épithète de fou, et traité comme tel. Au point de vue psychiatrique et juridique, l'enfant anormal n'est cependant pas un fou et on ne devrait pas faire peser sur lui la tare de l'internement. La création de ce service ouvert, qui sera un hôpital-école, rebutera moins les familles, en leur permettant à la fois de faire soigner leurs enfants malades et de leur faire donner l'éducation nécessaire. [...] L'organisation de ce service sera médico-administrative et je nomme Directrice responsable Mlle le docteur PASCAL, déjà médecin-chef du Service des femmes à l'asile d'aliénés de CHÂLONS, qui a une longue expérience de la psychologie morbide des enfants; cette nomination n'entraînera aucune dépense supplémentaire.

J'ai l'honneur, Monsieur le Ministre, de soumettre à votre ratification la création de ce service ouvert pour les enfants anormaux du Département de la Marne, que je serais heureux de pouvoir faire fonctionner dans un délai aussi rapproché que possible.[12]

[I am pleased to inform you that I have decided to create a special service in the Marne *Département* for handicapped children. The General Council approved this decision on 12 September 1922 and has committed the funding required. There is, indeed, no institution in the *département* specifically for handicapped children, in which

12 The Prefect, J. Brisac, DCAP Archives de la Marne (8 November 1922).

> they can be both cared for and educated; at present, mentally disabled children are sent away to other *départements* for the medical-pedagogic treatment they need if they are to develop. [...]
>
> This new service, a genuine medico-pedagogical Institute, will provide for two categories of handicapped children under sixteen:
>
> 1. boys and girls who are curable, or at least capable of improvement and social adaptation, and who are thus able to benefit from the provisions of the Education Act of 15 April 1909;
> 2. boys and girls who are uneducable and incapable of social adaptation – the dead weight of society: epileptics, psychopaths, imbeciles, idiots or sufferers from cerebral and medullary disorders – for whom constant care is needed.
>
> You will doubtless agree with me that these children, who constitute no danger to public safety, do not belong under the provisions of the Law of 1838 and that in consequence, this special service should be an open service. [...] In the present state of welfare for the handicapped, a backward child is stigmatized by being labelled 'mad' and treated as such. Yet, from the psychiatric and legal point of view, handicapped children are not mad and internment is a quite inappropriate burden on them. The creation of this open service, in the form of a hospital-school, will be less off-putting for families, for it will allow them to have their sick children treated and also given the education they need. [...] The organization of this service will be medico-administrative and I have appointed as Director Dr Pascal, currently *médecin-chef* in the women's section of the Châlons Asylum; she has many years of experience in treating morbid psychological conditions in children. [...]
>
> I herewith submit for your ratification the creation of this open service for handicapped children of the Marne Département, which I hope to establish in as short a time as possible.]

Paul Strauss, now minister for Public Health and reforming Radical Senator, had, both in his former profession as a journalist and throughout his political career, campaigned on welfare issues, particularly in relation to disadvantaged children.[13] He represented the progressive thinking of the day on the care and education of children with learning difficulties and, replying to Brisac, he approved Pascal's scheme:

> J'ai l'honneur de vous faire connaître que le principe de cette création me semble excellent; toutefois, je considère qu'il n'est pas possible de réunir dans un Pavillon dépendant de l'asile d'aliénés, les arriérés mentaux éducables pour lesquels la loi du 15 avril 1909 a prévu

13 Jean Jolly, *Dictionnaire des parlementaires français* (Paris: Presses Universitaires de France, 1966–77).

> la création de classes de perfectionnement. Il semble que seuls pourraient être justiciables du service ouvert projeté les mineurs épileptiques, idiots, crétins, anormaux inéducables, en un mot tous ceux qui trouvent leur place dans les quartiers spécialisés des asiles d'aliénés. Les anormaux de la 1ere catégorie pourraient au contraire être placés dans un Service spécial, absolument distinct de l'asile.[14]
>
> [I write to inform you that the principle [*of open services for handicapped children*] seems to me excellent. However, I believe that it is not possible to bring the educable mentally handicapped, for whom the law of 15 April 1909 provides for basic classes, into a wing directly attached to the asylum. In my opinion, the planned open clinic (*service ouvert*) would only be suitable for minors who are epileptics, idiots, cretins or uneducable – in a word, all those whose place is in the specialized sections of insane asylums. Abnormal children in the first category could, by contrast, be placed in a Special School, completely separate from the asylum.]

Strauss's letter reflects two major concerns in psychiatric reforms and more broadly the influence of the mental hygiene movement during the Third Republic: the first is that of *service ouvert*, the treatment of psychiatric patients in clinics, rather than having them interned in hospital, pioneered by Édouard Toulouse, and the second is the identification and education of so-called abnormal children as part of a growing interest in child psychology.[15] Toulouse, *médecin-chef* at the Sainte Anne Asylum, a fervent republican and sexual egalitarian, believed scientists should be at the forefront of the creation of a rational society, and opened the first public, open psychiatric service on 16 June 1922, the same year as Pascal's initiative at Châlons. The open clinic avoided the need to section patients, allowing the diagnosis and treatment of the less seriously ill in a clinical setting, but without the stigmatising recourse to internment in hospital.[16] The cost of treatment was covered by the law of 1893 which guaranteed medical assistance for all citizens. Though Pascal does not mention Toulouse by name in her correspondence, she would have been influenced by him on the issue of open services, particularly in the argument that they provided an opportunity for early diagnosis, before a patient was so ill as to require internment. We have seen in

14 Corr Paul Strauss & Prefect of the Marne, Asile Départemental d'Aliénés de Châlons-sur-Marne, Châlons DACP, AM (30 November 1922).

15 Ohayon, *IR*, 14–31.

16 Huteau, *Psychologie*, 69–140; Thomas, 'Open services', 131–154; Ohayon, *IR*, 31.

Chapter IV that at Prémontré Pascal had emphasized the need for early diagnosis, before the onset of more serious illness.[17]

The 1920s saw a growth in child psychology, behaviourism and collective psychology with the work of psychologists like Piaget, Binet and le Bon.[18] The Third Republic's commitment to educating French children in the values of republican citizenship, within a lay or non-clerical environment, led to efforts to diagnose children's potential at an early stage of development. Psychologists undertook scientific testing of children for sight and hearing on the grounds that any problem with these senses might affect comprehension. In a statistical study of the visual and auditory capacities of school children published in 1924, the author estimates that 20% of primary school children suffered from visual or auditory impairment and recommended universal testing to allow for early intervention.[19]

Thus, when it opened on 18 July 1923, Pascal's *Institut médico-pédagogique,* as it came to be called, formed part of a growing interest in child psychology and development. The originality of Pascal's initiative lay in her commitment to treating and, where possible, teaching severely handicapped children as part of the community, though in an environment in close proximity to the hospital. Children who formerly would have been confined in asylums were to be taught by state-trained teachers. She recognized the need to maintain close family links, insisting that her institute should serve the children of the Marne region and she travelled all over France to find and bring back to Châlons children who had been consigned to far-flung provincial asylums.[20]

Detailed arrangements for the new *Institut médico-pédagogique* were presented to the *Conseil Général* of the Marne at its September meeting of 1923. The Prefect, Jules Brisac, noted with approval that (1) the children would be selected under the rules for welfare assistance and were therefore not subject to the 1838 law on internment – hence it could be an 'open service'; (2) places at the Institute would be reserved, in the first instance, for children of the Marne region; (3) Dr Pascal was to be in charge of the medical side of the establishment;

17 Corr CP & Lenoir, Prémontré DACP (25 September 1921).

18 Ohayon, *IR*, 14–25.

19 Foucault [no initial given], 'Etude statistique', *Journal de psychologie normale et pathologique* (1924), 219–35.

20 Gordon, *French psychiatry*, 171–72; Henri Gaillac, *Les Maisons de correction 1830–1945* (Paris: Éditions Cujas, 1971); Georges Heuyer, *Enfants anormaux et délinquants juvéniles* (Paris: Seinheil, 1914); Corr CP & Prefect, Département of the Seine, Châlons DACP, AM (4 May 1930).

and (4) there would be an independent budget for the Institute, separate from that of the asylum. This financial autonomy was a crucial factor in the project's success.

Pascal submitted a detailed proposal describing the projected workings and management of the Institute. The buildings consisted of two wings, separating the children from adult patients, while the school contained separate quarters for boys and girls. Washing, toilet facilities and electric lighting were installed; cleaning and redecoration undertaken. A separate entrance from the rest of the hospital gave the new clinic physical independence from the asylum, comparable to its financial independence. The only thing that was lacking, but was planned for the future, was a parlour for visiting families. The boys' dormitory numbered forty-five beds, the girls' thirty.

These material arrangements, especially the physical separation of the asylum from Pascal's Institute, would avoid stigmatizing the children with the stain of compulsory internment, one of the principal impulses behind the concept of '*service ouvert*'. She wrote to the Prefect:

> Votre idée humanitaire d'avant-garde permettra à l'Institut médico-pédagogique d'être considéré comme un véritable hôpital-école, où les enfants déshérités et déjà si malheureux, recevront à la fois les soins nécessaires à leur organisme défectueux, et l'éducation en rapport avec leurs capacités intellectuelles, professionnelles et morales.
>
> [Your advanced and humanitarian idea will permit the *Institut médico-pédagogique* to be recognized as a genuine hospital-school, where deprived children, who have been through so much in their lives, will be able to receive both the care needed for their faulty bodies and the education appropriate to their intellectual, professional and moral capacities].[21]

A Mme Cellier was appointed as teacher for the 'educable' children. The remainder, needing additional care, were transferred to the children's wing of the asylum under Pascal's supervision.

Pascal's efforts attracted commendations from the authorities. M. Barchat, a member of the General Council, conveyed the inspectors' congratulations on the success of her initiative:

> Je saisis l'occasion qui m'est offerte pour adresser à Mlle le Docteur Pascal, créatrice et animatrice de l'Institut médico-pédagogique, nos félicitations et nos remerciements les plus chaleureux pour le

21 Corr CP & Prefect of the Marne (Jules Brisac), Châlons DACP, AM (18 July 1923).

> dévouement si éclairé qu'elle a bien voulu donner à cette œuvre d'une si haute portée sociale et humanitaire.[22]

> [I am seizing this opportunity to convey to Mlle Pascal, the creator and organizer of the *Institut médico-pédagogique*, our congratulations and heartfelt thanks for the enlightenment and dedication she has given to this work, which is of such importance to society and humanity in general.]

Each summer, the Institute mounted a gala celebration to mark the children's progress, celebrate their achievements and distribute prizes. The fête of August 1925 commemorated in the *Journal de la Marne*, comprised recitations, dramatic skits, singing by the children and musical performances by the staff. Jeanne Pascal, then nine years old, took part in a scene from Molière. The event was reported like a society garden party, hosted by Mlle la Doctoresse Pascal:

> Nous étions conviés, hier après-midi, à assister à la distribution des prix aux enfants de l'Institut médico-pédagogique. Pour cette cérémonie, une scène toute fleurie et enguirlandée est dressée en plein air, sous de magnifiques ombrages. Mlle la doctoresse Pascal, directrice de l'Institut, reçoit les invités avec une exquise amabilité.[23]

> [Yesterday afternoon we were invited to the distribution of prizes to the children of the *Institut médico-pédagogique*. For this ceremony, a stage decked with flowers and garlands had been set up in the open air, in the shade of magnificent trees. Dr Pascal, the Director of the Institute, received her guests with exquisite courtesy.]

After the programme of entertainments, all the children received prizes for their efforts during the year with encouragement to improve in the future. This fête, orchestrated and organized by Pascal, served to publicize the achievements of the children and the staff and to normalize the school in relation to the surrounding community. Newspaper coverage enabled her to make known to the outside world the work undertaken by the asylum with children who were often social rejects. In the words of the reporter: 'Il nous faut rendre hommage à celles qui se consacrent à ses pauvres enfants, déshérités de la vie' [We must pay homage to the ladies who devote themselves to these poor children, who have been deprived of so much in life].

One can glean something of Pascal's emotional commitment to the Institute's socially and educationally reforming purpose from a

22 Extract from the *Procès-verbal des délibérations du Conseil Général*, 27 May 1924, Châlons DACP, AM.

23 Anon, *Journal de la Marne* (August 1925).

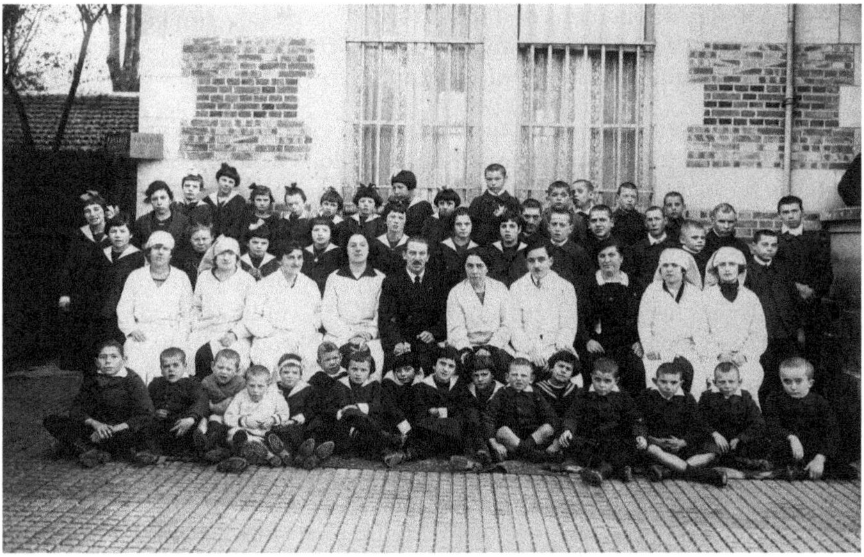

Fig 6. Children of the Institut médico-pédagogique with staff in the second row. Châlons sur Marne c. 1925

correspondence in 1930 concerning the subsequent fate of her project. On 16 April 1930, Georges Heuyer,[24] a leading child psychologist, wrote to Jules Brisac – now Director of the Office of Social Hygiene, an organization concerned with improving public health – to solicit his aid and influence for the education of severely handicapped children:

> Lorsque vous étiez Préfet de la MARNE, vous avez créé avec Mlle le Docteur PASCAL un institut médico-pédagogique à CHÂLONS qui eut rapidement une notoriété légitime car il répondait à un besoin incontestable et il donnait d'excellents résultats. Je crois que depuis votre départ et le départ de Mlle PASCAL, cet institut périclite. Or, il me paraît impossible de laisser quasi inutilisée une institution qui répond à des besoins immédiats et, qui, loin d'être vide, peut être remplie d'un jour à l'autre par des arriérés éducables, perfectibles et utilisables.
>
> Puisque vous avez eu, avec Mlle le docteur PASCAL l'excellente idée de créer cet institut, je fais appel à vous pour que vous preniez l'initiative de le faire réorganiser, au besoin même de le déplacer et de faire à CHÂLONS ou à REIMS une école de perfectionnement qui

24 For an assessment of Georges Heuyer (1884–1977) and his importance for neuro-psychiatric work with children see Ohayon, *L'Impossible Rencontre*, 173–84 and Henri Baruk, *La Psychiatrie française de Pinel à nos jours* (Paris: Presses Universitaires Françaises, 1967), 85–124.

serait le développement de l'Institut médico-pédagogique que vous aviez créé. Il a une utilité immédiate. Je me charge de faire la sélection des enfants qui y seront admis, les candidats ne manquent pas.[25]

[When you were Prefect of the Marne you created, together with Dr Pascal, a medico-pedagogic institute at Châlons which rapidly became deservedly famous, for it met an undoubted need and produced excellent results. I understand that since your departure and that of Mlle Pascal, this institute is collapsing. Yet it seems to me unthinkable that such an institution should be left virtually unused when it meets such urgent needs and, far from being empty, could be filled without delay with mentally handicapped but educable and useful children.

Since you, with Dr Pascal, were the originator of the excellent idea of creating this institute, I am appealing to you to take the initiative of reorganising it – if necessary, moving it, and setting up a training school in Châlons or Reims which would be a further development of the medico-pedagogic institute you founded. It would be of use straight away. I can take responsibility for choosing the children to be admitted; there is no lack of suitable candidates.]

Heuyer's recognition of Pascal's work was not replicated in Châlons after her departure. The new director instituted a policy which was contrary in almost every respect to what Pascal had inaugurated. She sent a passionate appeal to one of the former hospital inspectors, Barchat, who had praised her pioneering efforts:

Partie depuis 1926, j'ai appris que, pour des raisons diverses, cette malheureuse école a été désorganisée dans son principe de base. Les enfants trop tarés, susceptible de soins bien plus que d'éducation pédagogique ont été renvoyés à la Rochelle; le directeur, médecin actuel, et l'institutrice n'ont gardé que les enfants qui ne leur donnaient aucun mal.[26]

[Having left in 1926, I have now learned that for a variety of reasons the basic principles of this unfortunate school have been disrupted. The most handicapped children, who need care more than pedagogic training, have been sent to La Rochelle; the current medical director and the teacher have only kept on those children who are no trouble to teach.]

The founding principle of her work was the grouping together of all the handicapped children of the Marne at Châlons, offering there the care they required and the education of which they were capable. Now these children were once again separated from their

25 Corr Georges Heuyer & Jules Brisac, Châlons DACP, AM (16 April 1930).

26 Corr CP & Barchat, Châlons DACP, AM (4 May 1930).

families. 'La Marne n'a pas pu les garder, leur trouver une petite place sous le soleil de leur propre foyer familial. C'est navrant! pénible! douloureux!' [The Marne has not found a way to keep them, to find them a little space in the sun close to their families. This is heart-breaking – distressing – painful]. The new Prefect, Langeron, Prefect from 1924 to 1929, had, according to Pascal, undone all the social reforms instituted by Brisac, depriving the Marne region's most vulnerable children of a much-needed facility. The irony was that she had recently been summoned to the Ministry of Hygiene to be congratulated on her ground-breaking work at Châlons and had had to point out that her innovations had completely unravelled since her departure. Whereas other French *départements* had founded institutes on the Châlons model, the Marne had regressed. Like Heuyer, she begged Barchat to campaign for a new *institut médico-pédagogique*, and to ask M. Brisac for funding. Pascal's bitterness at the dissolution of her cherished institute is evident: 'On a oublié mon travail et mon dévouement; je veux le silence. Mais que l'Institut vive en dépit de la méchanceté des ingrats et de l'indifférence de ceux qui en avaient la charge' [My work and my dedication have been forgotten. I prefer to pass over that in silence. But the Institute deserves to live on, in spite of the malice of ungrateful people and the indifference of those in charge of it].[27]

Neither Heuyer's nor Pascal's letters seem to have borne fruit, as indicated by her glacial reply of 2 March 1931 to Langeron conveying apologies for not attending a meeting of the *Conseil d'Administration* of the *Institut médico-pédogogique*, remarking that apart from the fact that her letter of invitation was addressed to a Monsieur Pascal, this was the first time in the five years she had been a member of the council, that she had been invited to attend:

> Je me permets d'ajouter, Monsieur le Préfet, que je ne méritais pas d'être éliminée d'une façon systématique des réunions du Conseil d'administration; mes Collègues de ce Conseil pourront vous dire le dévouement désintéressé dont j'ai fait preuve pour organiser l'École d'anormaux de la Marne. Il aurait été plus juste de me laisser un peu de contact avec cette œuvre qui m'est toujours très chère.[28]
>
> [I wish to add that I did not deserve to be systematically removed from the meetings of the *Conseil d'Administration*; my colleagues on that committee can inform you of the disinterested dedication with which I ran the School for Handicapped Children in the Marne. It

27 Corr CP & Barchat, Châlons DACP, AM (4 May 1930).

28 Corr CP & Préfet de la Marne, Châlons DACP, AM (4 March 1931).

would have been fairer to leave me a little contact with this project to which I am still devoted.]

Though it is perhaps not surprising that Pascal should have been excluded from plans for her Institute once she no longer had direct responsibility for it, her sense of betrayal was strong and justified. She mourned the destruction of her plans and feared for the future of the children she had cared for. It might have been some consolation to her to know that the title *Institut* [or 'Centre'] *médico-pédagogique* remains in France for special schools for children with severe learning and motor difficulties and that at least one, part of the *Centre hospitalier de Sambre-Avesnois*, bears her name: *Centre médico-pédagogique Constance Pascal*. As far as Châlons was concerned, however, it would appear that a shift in the political climate and a lack of interest on the part of the new *médecin-chef* had resulted in the effective dismemberment of Pascal's project. Her ground-breaking initiative was largely forgotten, as we note in Henri Baruk's omission of her name in a discussion of research into infantile neuro-psychiatry, where he lists such figures as Binet, Heuyer and Simon, presumably not aware that Pascal, whom he had earlier noted for her outstanding work on *dementia praecox*, had also contributed, as Heuyer had recognized, to child psychiatry.[29]

Another key event for Pascal in 1924 was her formal adoption of Jeanne, now seven years old. Since 1804, the civil code had prohibited child adoption, only allowing adults over fifty to adopt other consenting adults. Anxieties about falling population, exacerbated by the bloodletting of the First World War, consequent social dislocation and the great number of war orphans, persuaded legislators of the desirability of change.[30] The law of 19 June 1923 under Article 343 permitted child adoption, provided that the adopter could show evidence of previous care for the child, that the adoptee would benefit both materially and morally and that the adopter was over forty years old. In 1924, Pascal was forty-seven. The law made no distinction between single and married persons wishing to adopt. Indeed single women adopting children were seen by some feminists as demonstrating women's growing independence.[31] From Pascal's point of view, although her daughter had no parental recognition in law (her birth certificate stating 'parents unknown' was never

29 Baruk, *La Psychiatrie française*, 85–104.

30 Ohayon, *IR*, 21.

31 Rachel G. Fuchs, *Contested Paternity: Constructing Families in Modern France* (Baltimore: John Hopkins University Press, 2008), 217–39; for the Adoption Law of 1923 see Dalloz, *Recueil périodique et critique* (1923), 257–62.

amended), adoption protected Jeanne's civil status and her rights to inheritance after her mother's death.

Whereas from 1915 to 1921 she had published relatively little, no doubt due to the double pressures of work in war-time conditions and her maternal preoccupations, at Châlons Pascal returned to her research. Her impressive publication record throughout her career (see the Bibliography in this volume) reflects a psychiatric culture in which published research was crucial to professional advancement. Like many of her colleagues, Pascal aspired to win a position in the Paris asylum system – *les Asiles de la Seine* – the only region to have its own *concours* and which in the highly centralized French system was the locus of prestige for her profession. Psychiatry, unlike general medicine, was a state-funded profession and managed as a branch of the French civil service. The typical employment pattern in psychiatry, as in state-funded education, was for a newly qualified candidate to begin his or her career with one or more postings in the provinces, with the ultimate goal of a Paris appointment. Pascal's increased research activity at Châlons probably reflected an effort to improve her professional profile, as part of her ambition to be appointed to the Paris region.

Between 1922 and 1926, Pascal published numerous articles and one monograph. Two publications will be discussed here: her sole-authored 'Syndrome Psychique Fondamental des Démences' and 'Chocs Emotionels Pathogènes et Thérapeutiques', written with a colleague, Jean Davesne.[32] Davesne was a native of Champagne and an intern at Châlons during Pascal's tenure there, when he became not only her colleague but, according to the Rees family, was treated by Pascal like an adopted son. When he later transferred to Maison Blanche, Davensne looked after Pascal following her operation for cancer in 1928, when he seems to have quarrelled with General Mengin. Relations between Davesne and his patroness cooled further

32 Communication from Margaret Rees (13 April 2003). The articles to be discussed here are Constance Pascal, 'Syndrome psychique fondamental des démences', *Journal de psychologie normale et pathologique* (1923); Constance Pascal and Jean Davesne, 'Chocs émotionnels pathogènes et thérapeutiques', *Journal de psychologie normale et pathologique* (1926). Other articles co-authored between 1922 and 1926 are: Constance Pascal and Jean Davesne, 'La psychiatrie d'urgence', *La Pratique médicale française* (1925); Constance Pascal and Jean Davesne, 'La thérapeutique sanguine dans les psychoses', *La Presse médicale* (1925); Constance Pascal and Jean Davesne, 'Les psychocolloïdoclasies: anaphylaxie mental spontanée', *La Presse médicale* (1925); Constance Pascal and Jean Davesne, 'Les abcès de fixation dans les psychoses', *Archives internationales de neurologie* (1926); Constance Pascal and Jean Davesne, *Traitement des maladies mentales par les chocs* (Paris: Masson, 1926).

when Pascal reproached him for neglecting his illegitimate child. Their collaboration in published works ceased after 1926.

The joint work of Pascal and Davesne appeared in a psychological, not a psychiatric, journal, which demonstrates a shift in Pascal's interests from a largely descriptive approach on *dementia praecox* to exploring her patients' subjectivity and the importance of affective memory in understanding mental illness.[33] In this she reflected a wider movement in psychology in France represented by Théodule Ribot, Pierre Janet, Georges Dumas, Alfred Binet and Henri Bergson on theories of the unconscious mind.[34] In 'Syndrome', while not dissenting from the predominant physiological model for the origin of dementia, thought to be lesions in the brain (citing Klippel and Lhermitte) Pascal follows Binet, Simon and Ribot in examining dementia as a dynamic mental process.[35] 'La démence est une inertie fonctionnelle et non la ruine définitive de la pensée, la destruction anatomique du cerveau' [Dementia is a functional inertia, not the definitive ruin of thought, the anatomical destruction of the brain] ('Syndrome', 148). The war had thrown up many examples of shell-shocked soldiers, whose mental traumas did not alter their brain function. Symptoms such as aphasia, formerly thought to signify material damage to the brain, were now considered instead a dynamic disturbance of nervous energy.

In her work of 1911 on *dementia praecox*, Pascal had remarked on the early loss of social feeling in patients suffering from the disease. The emphasis of psychiatrists in the past on a patient's degree of intellectual function as a diagnostic tool had led, she believed, to the neglect of states of feeling and their primacy in forming the human personality. When the affective sphere is compromised, the whole personality crumbles:

> La sphère affective avec ses tendances, ses désirs et ses sentiments participe à la constitution du moi dynamique et à l'organisation du

33 The three major psychological journals of the period were Théodule Ribot's *Revue philosophique*, with a focus on scientific psychology, *L'année psychologique* and the *Journal de psychologie normale et pathologique*. They emphasized experimental research based on medical models. Ohayon, *IR*, 14–25.

34 Thomas Hardy Leahey, *A History of Psychology: Main Currents in Psychological Thought* (Upper Saddle River, New Jersey: Prentice Hall, 2000), 230–36.

35 Klippel and J. Lhermitte, 'Les démences, anatomie, pathologie et pathogénie', *Revue de psychiatrie* (1905), 485–518; Théodule Ribot, *Les Maladies de la personnalité* (Paris: Alcan, 1895); Alfred Binet and Théodore Simon, 'Nouvelle théorie psychologique et clinique de la démence', *L'Année Psychologique* (1909), 168–272. Baruk cites Pascal's monograph on *dementia praecox*, based on Kraeplin's anatomical model, as definitive.

moi statique. Évocatrice, sélectrice, inhibitrice, elle est la fonction de la cohésion mentale. Conservatrice, elle assure la stabilité des souvenirs et des croyances. Si l'intelligence et la volonté sont le plus beau fruit de la personnalité humaine, elles n'en sont pas la racine; elles nous donnent notre valeur, elles ne constituent pas notre fond ('Syndrome', 150–51).

[The affective sphere, with its leanings, desires and feelings, plays a part in building the dynamic self and in organising the static self. Evoking, selecting, inhibiting, it is the very function of mental cohesion. It conserves memories and beliefs, assuring their stability. The intelligence and the will may be the finest fruits of the human personality, but they are not its roots; they give us our value but they do not constitute our foundations.]

To lose our capacity for feeling is to lose ourselves:

La mémoire des sentiments est une partie du moi qui demeure une et continue sous le flux des variations incessantes et assure notre identité; elle est la base de tous nos devoirs et de toutes nos responsabilités; l'amnésie affective, c'est l'oubli de notre identité, c'est l'oubli de nous-mêmes. ('Syndrome', 150–51).

[The memory of feelings is that part of the self that remains unaltered through the flux of perpetual change and ensures our identity; it is the basis of our whole sense of duty and responsibility; to have amnesia in the affective sphere is to forget one's identity; to forget who one is.]

To contemporary readers, Pascal's discussion of affective memory, that is to say, the recollection not of events or facts but of the colouration, the seeming re-experience of a past state, is redolent of Proust's involuntary memory. Later, in *Chagrins d'amour et psychoses* (1935), she would distinguish between the retrieval of a lost past in Proust's writing and the haunting memories of trauma which patients are unable to forget or exorcize. Here in 'Syndrome', as Barbier argues, she credits Freud with the idea that a partial discharge of emotion can lead to the creation of psychoses representing unsatisfied emotions, which emerge by disguising themselves as metaphors, symbols, morbid dreams, delirium or esoteric language:[36]

C'est le mérite de l'école de Freud d'avoir montré ces décharges partielles, ces déguisements nombreux qui trompent la censure. C'est son tort de n'avoir pas compris le jeu de sensibilisation et de désensibilisation émotionnelle du psychisme. [...] Ainsi, lorsqu'un

36 Barbier, *VOCP*, 109.

patient succombe dans la psychose, c'est parce qu'il a perdu le moyen de se désensibiliser, il fléchit sous la surcharge émotionnelle.[37]

[It is to the credit of the Freudian school that it revealed these partial discharges, whose many disguises deceive the censor. It was wrong, however, in failing to understand the workings of emotional sensitization and desensitization of the psyche. [...] Thus, when a patient falls into psychosis, it is because he has lost the means of desensitizing himself; he gives way under an excess of emotion.]

Pascal's interest in affective memory and the emotions followed the work of Ribot and Paulhan, who studied unconscious mental states and automatic memory patterns in the context of mental illness. Already in 1895, taking a firmly materialist and evolutionary position, Ribot argued that our personality, our sense of self, has its roots in the biological organism located in the brain and nervous system, which constitute the real personality.

L'encéphale est comme un laboratoire plein de mouvement où mille travaux se font à la fois. La cérébration inconsciente, n'étant pas soumise à la condition du temps, ne se faisant pour ainsi dire dans l'espace, peut agir dans plusieurs endroits à la fois. La conscience est l'étroit guichet par où une toute petite partie de ce travail nous apparaît (Ribot, *Maladies de la mémoire*, 26–27).

[The encephalon is like a busy laboratory in which a thousand activities are going on at once. Unconscious mental processes, which are not under the sway of time but occur, as it were only in space, may operate in several places at once. Consciousness is the narrow window through which a very small part of this work is made visible to us.]

The conscious mind, Ribot thought, is only partly aware of the sum total of knowledge in the biological organism. The conscious self is therefore a small part of the entire psychic personality. He suggested that affective memory was not an illusion, as some psychologists thought, or a new feeling attached to an old image, but a genuine reliving of the past. At rare moments the past as it was experienced may be reawakened in us. Odours, in particular, can elicit a state of feeling, a fundamental memory clearly related to childhood:

Cet état affectif a été éprouvé plusieurs fois pendant mon enfance, un très petit nombre de fois ou jamais depuis. Il avait disparu complètement de ma synthèse personnelle et il apparaît avec un

37 CP & Jean Davesne, *Le Traitement des maladies mentales par les chocs* (Paris: Masson, 1926), 68.

> air étrange, vieillot. En même temps qu'il apparaît, je sens que c'est quelque chose d'ancien et d'oublié. De plus, son apparition est fugace, j'ai besoin de le retenir, ce n'est pas un état stable; il n'est aucunement en rapport avec mon état actuel; il apparaît comme un anachronisme véritable [...] La durée de ces évocations a toujours été de quelques secondes à peine, puis venaient les souvenirs intellectuels évoqués par cette orientation brusque, d'origine affective, vers des périodes d'enfance. Il me semble qu'il y a là une preuve indéniable de l'existence de la mémoire affective.[38]
>
> [I experienced this affective state several times in my childhood but rarely or never since. It had completely vanished from my personal mental makeup and now carries a strange, outdated feeling. As I feel it surfacing, it appears like something ancient and forgotten. What's more, its appearance is fleeting, I have to try and hold it back, it is not stable, it bears no relation to my present state of mind, but seems a true anachronism [...] These evocations have only ever lasted a couple of seconds, and what follow are the intellectual memories evoked by this sudden emotional turn towards the days of childhood. This seems to me to offer undeniable proof of the existence of affective memory.]

Frédéric Paulhan also explored the concept of affective – or emotional (as distinct from intellectual) – memory. This idea of the retrieval of what something felt like or how it was experienced was developed, as we have noted, most famously in fiction by Proust. Psychologists like Ribot and Paulhan, whom Proust very possibly read, were interested in moving away from the psychiatric staple of pure outward description of mental states, nosology, towards attempting to unravel and at the same time validate subjective experience.[39] Paulhan recalls in a passage that conjures up *À la recherche du temps perdu*:

38 Ribot, *Problèmes de la psychologie affective* (1910), 46–47, quoting Pierron, *Revue philosophique* II (March 1907).

39 The extent of Proust's reading in and indebtedness to contemporary psychology is not entirely clear. However according to Jean-Yves Tadié, *Marcel Proust, Biographie* (Paris: Gallimard, 1996), 105, Proust's parents thought he suffered from 'la maladie de la volonté' [infirmity of the will], one of Ribot's diagnostic categories. More broadly Proust was widely read in the philosophy and psychology of the day. Probable influences in psychology were Théodule Ribot, Frédéric Paulhan and Pierre Janet. 'Proust's theories – philosophical and psychological – are reflections of the intellectual spirit of the times', Jack Jordan, 'The Unconscious', *The Cambridge Companion to Proust*, Richard Bales, ed. (Cambridge: Press Syndicate of the University of Cambridge, 2001), 102.

> Il arrive assez souvent que je sens se lever tout à coup en moi des impressions se rapportant à mon enfance, à ma première jeunesse, impressions depuis longtemps disparues, qui ne correspondent plus guère à mon moi d'aujourd'hui. Des souvenirs, ou bien la similitude de certaines circonstances extérieures, un village retrouvé après une longue absence, un livre lu jadis et mis à l'écart ensuite, la ressemblance même très vague d'un paysage, d'une maison, une photographie, mille circonstances diverses éveillent de temps en temps des sentiments, ravivent des émotions qui se rapportent à un moi qui n'est plus le mien (Paulhan, *Fonction de la mémoire*, 3).
>
> [It quite often happens that I find impressions from my childhood suddenly rising up within me, impressions from infancy that have long since disappeared and bear little relation to the self I am today. It may be a memory, or it may be the similarity of some external circumstance, a village revisited after a long absence, a book read long ago and never opened since, the resemblance, however vague, of a landscape or a house or a photograph – a whole range of different circumstances can awaken these occasional feelings and bring to life emotions belonging to an earlier self that is no longer mine.]

Whereas Paulhan's and Ribot's focus is on the sense that the affective memory relates to a vanished time and self, in Paulhan's phrase, 'impressions from infancy that [...] bear little relation to the self I am today', for Pascal the affective memory reveals a constant of personality and performs a co-ordinating function of our multiple selves in time. In dementia, the first stage in mental disintegration, according to Pascal, is the loss of affective capacity, feeling for others, followed eventually by loss of will and finally of intellect. She argues that all forms of dementia are similar in their effects even though they may be provoked by different causes:

> La perte du contact affectif constitue, avec l'amnésie des sentiments, les signes fondamentaux de premier ordre de la démence. Le persécuté vit en conflit avec son milieu; le maniaque est en contact perpétuel avec le monde extérieur; *le dément est étranger à son ambiance*. L'unité de la personnalité est maintenue et réglée par le contact affectif avec la réalité qui l'entoure. [...] La perte du contact affectif isole le malade du monde extérieur, le présent réel disparaît, les événements ne laissent plus de trace, la notion de la durée disparaît avant celle de l'espace ('Syndromes', 152–53).
>
> [Two things constitute the fundamental sign of the first stage of dementia: amnesia of the feelings and the loss of emotional contact. The paranoiac lives in conflict with his milieu; the maniac is in constant contact with the outside world; *the demented patient is a stranger to his own surroundings*. Unity of the personality is maintained

> and controlled by affective contact with surrounding reality. [...] The loss of affective contact cuts off the patient from the outside world, present reality fades away, events no longer leave a trace, he loses the sense of time before that of space.]

Pascal's descriptions of dementia, whether senile dementia, schizophrenia (*dementia praecox*) or general paralysis (syphilitic dementia), are based on a dynamic biological model. Although dementia follows a destructive path in the dissolution of personality, the 'morbid process' is uncertain in its development and may allow remissions. From the perspective of therapeutic intervention, this dynamic, functional theory of psychobiology offers hope for the alleviation of symptoms if not of cure, whereas the degeneracy model does not. She insists that the capacity for feeling rather than the rational Cartesian intellect constitutes the core of the human personality: 'La démence, quelle qu'en soit la cause, est toujours un processus d'involution affective; la décadence intellectuelle est subordonnée à la lésion de l'affectivité' ('Syndrome', 156) [Dementia, whatever its cause, always consists of an inward-turning of the emotions; the corruption of the intellect is less important than the injury to affectivity].

In 'Syndrome', Pascal does not examine causal influences, but focuses on the similarities in mental dissolution in dementia. However in 'Chocs émotionnels, pathogènes et thérapeutiques' (1926), Pascal and Davesne examine the effects of trauma or shocks, arguing that they may precipitate mental illness as well as provide a potential means of cure. 'Chocs' reviews the theoretical and experimental work on shock therapy, developed more fully in her monograph, published jointly with Davesne, *Le traitement des maladies mentales par les chocs* (1926). Pascal's experimentation with various forms of shock therapy in the 1920s and 30s was part of a wider movement in psychiatry to find cures, or at least alleviation, for conditions that had formerly been thought of as inherited, incurable and degenerative mental diseases.[40] Shorter and Healy credit Pascal with introducing the word 'shock' to French psychiatry in 1926, providing an over-

40 For the history of shock therapies see Max Fink, 'Induced seizures and human behaviour', *Psychobiology of Convulsive Therapy*, eds. Max Fink, and others (Washington D C: V.H. Winston, 1974); Max Fink, 'Meduna and the origins of convulsive therapy', *American Journal of Psychiatry*, 141: 9 (1984), 1034–39; Renato M. E. Sabbatini, 'The History of shock therapy in psychiatry', *Brain and Mind Magazine* (December and March 1997–98); Edward Shorter and David Healy, *Shock Therapy: the History of Electroconvulsive Treatment in Mental Illness* (New Jersey: Rutgers University Press, 2007), 4–10.

arching rationale for its use, and they quote her attack on psychiatric fatalism:

> To have to look on helplessly at the fatal advance of psychosis is just to endorse fate; accepting the predisposition to delusions and the fatal destiny of constitution also means renouncing the practical applications of the biological sciences that have modified the study of general pathology (*Shock Therapy*, 4).

The two models of intervention followed were biological and psychological, the latter epitomized by, but not limited to, Freudian psychoanalysis. With regard to the biological model, European psychiatrists from 1917 to the late 1930s experimented with a range of physiological shocks, among them malaria-induced fever, insulin-induced coma and convulsions, metrazol-induced convulsions and, in 1937, electroconvulsive shock therapy. Beginning with the observation that few epileptics suffered from *dementia praecox* and that few patients with *dementia praecox* were epileptics, the inference was drawn that convulsions and mental illness were incompatible. Further, the observation that psychosis in some patients improved after a high fever led Wagner-Jauregg in Vienna, for example, to inject patients with malarial blood to provoke a fever shock. Biological shock treatments marked the inter-war period of therapeutic optimism.[41]

Constance Pascal's place in this highly experimental phase of treatment of severe mental illnesses is indicative not only of the psychiatric fashions of the time, but of her originality. She did not accept uncritically the biological model as the only therapeutic mode of treatment, as is shown by her interest in Freud and her experience of trauma, stemming from observations of shell-shocked soldiers. Against this she laid equal weight on patients' life experience. It followed that while she performed physiological experiments on them, she also experimented with 'emotional shocks;' a version of psycho-therapy if not Freudian psychoanalysis. Never abandoning a materialist position, she shared the hope that patients were not condemned forever by their illness due to their hereditary make-up, but that neurological changes to overcome mental illness could be effected in a variety of ways. Though devoted to the care and possible cure of her patients, she – in common with most of the psychiatric profession – carried out experiments of undoubted mental and physical severity on patients who could not possibly give consent.

'Chocs' exemplifies the experimental, therapeutic enthusiasm of the period. It aims to analyse and interpret emotional syndromes

41 Fink, 'Induced Seizures', 2.

in the light of modern biological knowledge, to trace the movement from the 'normal' to the pathological, to distinguish morbid emotion from healthy, therapeutic emotion.[42] This effort to interpret emotional syndromes relates directly to Pascal's interest in the relation of the emotions to memory and their function in maintaining the social personality:

> L'émotion est le phénomène le plus vivant et le plus agissant du psychisme mouvant; grâce à elle, l'intelligence se rythme sur les vibrations de la vie organique. Son action triple: psychologique, physiologique et biologique, fait d'elle un facteur puissant de création, de destruction et de restauration. [...] Il est nécessaire, dans l'intérêt de la thérapeutique des maladies mentales et surtout du traitement par les chocs, qui a une application déterminée, d'essayer d'apprécier son influence exclusive sur les syndromes émotionnels et d'étudier le choc émotionnel thérapeutique ('Chocs', 457).

> [Emotion is the most vital and active part of the dynamic psyche; it is what allows the intelligence to follow the rhythms of organic life. Its triple function – psychological, physiological and biological – makes it a powerful agent of creation, destruction and rehabilitation. [...] In the interests of therapy in mental illness, and especially shock treatment, which has a specific application, we must try to understand the importance of the direct influence of these treatments on emotional syndromes and study the therapeutic effects of emotional shock techniques.]

Popular language commonly sees the influence of emotional upheavals as a primary cause of illness, a common-sense perception often acknowledged by psychiatrists, who nonetheless, Pascal and Davesne suggest, have not attempted to find causal links between emotional shocks and mental troubles. The dominance of degeneracy theory in nineteenth and early twentieth-century psychiatry lay behind this neglect of precipitating traumas as the assumption was that mental degeneration was (1) incurable and (2) had its origins, not in an event, but in an inherited disorder.[43] Dynamic psychology, the authors argue, derived from psycho-biology and psychoanalysis has focused on the role of the emotions in certain psychoses. Static conceptions of the personality in traditional psychiatry, based on predispositions, or inevitable morbidity, are now superseded by

42 Pascal and Davesnes, 'Chocs', 451.

43 Dowbiggin, *Inheriting Madness*, 1–2.

active psychotherapy and shock treatments to desensitize a morbid sensibility.[44]

The shell-shocked victims thrown up by the Great War, thought initially by many psychologists to be shirkers or subject to auto-suggestion, had provided medical literature with a rich range of observations, in which emotional states predominate.[45] In 'Chocs' it is assumed that emotional war wounds have a physiological equivalent:

> La guerre d'usure a créé une usure psychique et organique. [...] Le manque de confort, l'insomnie, le conflit des prérogatives, les frictions de la promiscuité, l'inaction, l'éloignement des siens, les deuils, les inquiétudes, l'ennui, le surmenage déterminé par les efforts répétés de la réaction (endurance, ténacité, patience), la sensation du risque, les accès de désespoir alternant avec la résignation, créent cet état de *pléthore de malaises* qui sensibilise progressivement le psychisme ('Chocs', 460–61).
>
> [The war of attrition also created psychological and organic attrition. [...] Lack of creature comforts, lack of sleep, conflicting prerogatives, the frustrations of overcrowding, inaction, homesickness, the death of comrades, anxiety, boredom, the stress brought about by the perpetual effort to react to circumstances with endurance, tenacity and patience, the sense of imminent danger, fits of despair alternating with resignation, all these problems cumulatively create a state of *multiple unease* which sensitizes the psyche.]

Soldiers who had shown great courage in battle were thrown into a panic over trifles. Reviewing numerous articles testifying to the extreme over-sensitivity exhibited by victims of trench warfare, Pascal and Davesne emphasize the disturbances to their physical systems (higher blood pressure, for example) as conclusive evidence of the reality and validity of shell shock. In an excursion into contemporary literature, Pascal cites Paul Bourget's novel *La Geôle* (1923), which features a protagonist with an allegedly hereditary tendency to suicide overcome by a powerful and traumatic familial revelation, as a dramatic example of the transformative power of emotion. Unlike Bourget, Pascal and Davesne do not abandon a materialist position in favour of Catholic conversion. But it was characteristic of Pascal, an omnivorous reader, to look for illustrations and parallels of unbalanced mental states in literature and philosophy.

Much of 'Chocs' is taken up with a description of the assumed mechanism of pathological emotion, both its physiological and

44 'Chocs', 456.

45 Ohayon, *IR*, 17–20.

psychological effects, described as a wave expending itself through the nervous system and following a determinable pattern ('Chocs', 463). The passages on *mémoire affective* or *souvenirs émotionnels* almost certainly reflect Pascal's own voice. An emotional charge, or trauma, may not exhaust itself but rather remain as an affective memory which, when recalled, can unleash psychosis. Pathological memories condemn individuals to perpetual recall – they are prisoners of their past. A quotation from Georges Bataille tellingly sums up the power of the past:

> Le passé est un second cœur qui bat en nous.
> Le passé n'est jamais tout à fait le passé.
> Non pas derrière nous comme on croît, mais devant.
> L'ombre de ce qui fut devant nous se projette.[46]
>
> [The past is a second heart beating within us
> The past is never entirely past
> It is not behind us, as we believe, but before us.
> The shadow of what has been is projected ahead of us.]

In this article, couched in technical and medical psychological language, Pascal nevertheless utilizes popular and literary examples of trauma and emotive memory because, as she argues, the positivist, scientific imagination fails to take account of the emotional reality of patients' mental disorders. While committed to scientific materialism, Pascal here embodies the views of 'romantic psychiatry', which held that the causes of mental illness lay in patients' psychological history, especially their emotional lives.[47]

Because emotional trauma was thought to leave physiological traces and pathological imbalances in a biochemical sense, psychiatrists experimented with a therapy based on counter-shocks. Janet had noted that confirmed neurotics could be cured by an unexpected catastrophe. Hysteria had been treated by 'shocks' long before Freudian psychoanalysis had emerged as one of many methods to exorcize memory via emotional shocks.[48] It is true that Freud himself did not apply his techniques to seriously psychotic patients but saw his model of the mind as having general validity, a view Pascal seems to have shared. As one of the early admirers of Freud in France, she was impressed by his accounts of freeing patients

46 Georges Bataille, 'Songe d'un soir d'amour', quoted in 'Chocs émotionnels', 467.

47 Leahey, *History of Psychology:*,234–5.

48 Naomi Segal, 'Witnessing through the skin: the hysteric's body as text', *Journal of Romance Studies*, 9: 3 (2009), 73–85.

from their repressed memories, but she became sceptical of his theory of sexual aetiology as the primary cause of mental illness. Like Freud she recognized the difficulty of treating severely ill psychiatric patients by the talking cure.[49] 'Si cette méthode thérapeutique est difficile à réaliser et ne réussit pas toujours, c'est qu'elle représente une méthode de désensibilisation spécifique; le psychanalyste doit trouver le complexe sexuel pathogène et provoquer sa décharge; toute autre désensibilisation est inutile' ('Chocs', 486) [If this therapeutic method is difficult to implement and does not always succeed, it is because it represents a specific method of desensitization: the psychoanalyst must find out the pathological sexual complex and cause it to discharge; any other form of desensitization is useless].

In the same year, 1926, Pascal and Davesne followed 'Chocs' with a monograph, *Le Traitement des maladies mentales par les chocs*. This work won the *Prix Ch. Boullard* of *l'Académie Nationale de Médecine*. The citation accompanying the prize is revealing of the ambitions and limitations of their therapeutic method. The commentator notes that the work displayed 'un désir fervent et ardent d'enrichir la thérapeutique jusqu'ici décevante des diverses psychoses, désir qui contraste avec les méthodes d'observation et d'expérimentation' [A fervent and ardent desire to enrich the hitherto disappointing results of therapy on various psychoses, a desire which contrasts with their methods of observation and experimentation].[50] He further comments that, though their work showed evidence of 'un esprit généreux' [a generous spirit], it had to be said that a fervent desire is not sufficient and that unambiguous results were rare.

Pascal and Davesne's monograph also received favourable recognition from a review in the *British Medical Journal*, which stressed the originality of their research within contemporary psychiatry:[51]

> In a volume entitled *Traitement des maladies mentales par les chocs,* Mlle C. Pascal and M. Jean Davesne record their extensive experience of the treatment of mental diseases by the introduction of a variety of different agents into the organism in an attempt to imitate the effects of inter-current disorders upon the psychoses. As every psychiatrist knows, these effects are sometimes remarkable, since a bodily illness, such as pneumonia or enteric fever, may bring about amelioration, or even a cure, of an apparently hopeless case of insanity. The authors have applied 'shock therapy' to a large number of patients, both acute

49 For Freud's reception in France see Ohayon, *IR*, 20–134.

50 Quoted in Barbier, *VOCP*, 111.

51 Anon, 'Shock-therapy in the psychoses', *The British Medical Journal* (29 January 1927), 194. I am indebted to Margaret Rees for this reference.

> and chronic. [...] At first the fixation abscess method, which consists in the provocation of a purulent focus by the subcutaneous injection of turpentine [...] subsequently, the following agents were utilized for injection: colloidal metals; peptones; vaccines; milk; nucleinate of soda; horse serum; and blood taken either from the patient himself, or from another patient in a state of remission. [...] The authors endeavour to explain the nature of the psychopathic constitution in biological terms as a profound humoral and neuro-vegation defect. The book is written in the spirit of hopefulness and enthusiasm, and the authors believe that the methods of investigation which they describe contain not only the principle of the cure of the chronic psychoses, but also their secret. We can recommend this original and interesting monograph to the attention of psychiatrists.

If Pascal and Davesne's ambition to move psychiatry in a firmly therapeutic direction was not at this stage matched by their results, their theoretical groundwork on the emotions was nevertheless recognized as an important, indeed ground-breaking, contribution to psychiatric literature.

'Chocs' would have resonance for Pascal in two directions. The first was to contribute to the new psychiatric interest in toxic shocks to the physical system in order to release or subdue pathological mental energy; the second was to study emotional trauma and its effects in creating psychosis, which culminated in her 1935 monograph, *Chagrins d'amour et psychoses*. Yet the bewildering and almost random array of shock therapies listed in the *British Medical Journal's* review raises troubling issues. The ethical vacuum in psychiatry in relation to toxic shock experiments on patients incapable of consent remains one of the most disturbing aspects of Pascal's work and that of psychiatry generally at this period, and this vacuum would partially contribute to the disasters befalling interned patients in France during the Vichy years.[52] In this regard, Shorter and Healy note: 'after World War II, her [Pascal's] enthusiasm for these particular injections was seen as horrific. Though Pascal brought the concept of "shock" to psychiatry, she did not mean it in the sense of convulsions, which she was at pains to avoid with her various therapies' (*Shock Therapy*, 10). The tensions visible in Pascal's work between, on the one hand, regarding her patients as experimental objects and, on the other, seeing them

52 C. Buvat-Pochon, *Les Traitements du choc d'autrefois en psychiatrie* (Paris: Librairie Le François, 1939). 'The dedication to this work is to Mlle le Docteur C. Pascal, in memoriam'; see also von Bueltzingsloeven, *HF*, 353–67 on French psychiatry and shock therapy and on psychiatric experiments with vitamin supplements for starving patients during World War II, 134–50.

as individual subjects – though characteristic of the profession as a whole – remained unresolved.

Pascal put her talent for publicity into efforts to enhance the profile of the mental health services, envisaging her psychiatric role as reaching well beyond the confines of the hospitals where she worked. She recognized the prejudice surrounding mental illness and the almost superstitious horror inspired by psychiatric hospitals in the public mind, which classified them, along with the prisons of the *Ancien Régime*, as sites of arbitrary detention. In a leading article in *Le Matin*, a moderate republican daily, she robustly defended the role of psychiatric hospitals to alleviate the suffering of patients, arguing, in this case, against criticisms of the potentially oppressive nature of the institution.[53] The current law, which provided for the sectioning of patients, incorporated in her view extensive safeguards against abuse: 'La loi de 1838 est à la fois une loi de protection sociale et une loi de protection individuelle' [The law of 1838 offers protection both for society and for the individual].[54] Nevertheless, the closed nature of asylums, the sometimes arbitrary nature of incarceration, and the public's fear of mental illness combined to make prejudice difficult to counteract.[55]

It was difficult to publicize reforms in psychiatric treatment, Pascal pointed out, whereas a violent attack on a member of the public by a psychiatric patient would receive enormous and unwelcome publicity:

> Les préjugés concernant la folie persistent avec une ténacité effroyable. Il suffit d'un incident dans les rues, un fou en liberté qui plante un couteau dans le dos d'un passant ou d'un scandale fâcheux dans un asile pour que les erreurs les plus moyenâgeuses basées toujours sur les faits exceptionnels sortent de l'ombre, se propagent et accaparent l'opinion publique.
>
> [Popular prejudice in relation to madness is appallingly persistent. It only takes one incident in the street, a madman at large who stabs a passer-by, or one unfortunate scandal in an asylum, for the most medieval attitudes, always based on exceptional circumstances, to come out of the woodwork, to be broadcast and take over public opinion.]

53 Charle, *Le Siècle de la presse*, 157–160.

54 Constance Pascal, 'Les asiles d'aliénés ne sont pas des geôles', *Le Matin* (12 February 1924).

55 Goldstein, *Console*, 322–77; Ripa, *Women and Madness*, 115–37.

In her defence of the law of 1838, Pascal was primarily interested in dispelling the prejudices surrounding asylums and the care of the mentally ill, and to emphasize the therapeutic and protective value of the asylum for the patient. Though she did not tackle here the wider criticisms of internment policy seen as potentially oppressive, her work at Châlons on open services for children had pointed in that direction. Indeed, her intervention was interpreted by the press as part of a reforming agenda: 'The afflicted people she treats are specially devoted to her and this is explainable [*sic*] when one reads one of her articles, "Asylums are no longer jails, but hospitals," she says, "and the insane are treated as sick people and no longer punished or demonised."'[56] Her subsequent interviews, given to journalists in the 1930s, aimed to open psychiatric hospitals to public scrutiny and to remove the pall of fear and mystery that hung over them.

Pascal left Châlons for Paris in 1925, achieving her long-held ambition to be appointed to an asylum in the capital. She departed not without reluctance, having to relinquish control over her school and children's services. Her nursing staff was disconsolate, writing a formal letter of farewell that conveyed their pride at Pascal's success and their concerns about their future without her:

> Les infirmières du Service des Femmes se permettent d'adresser à leur Médecin Chef, leurs sincères félicitations. Elles ont appris avec plaisir, le succès qu'il a remporté à un concours difficile, où sa science a pu triompher si facilement. Sur leur joie, passe une vague de tristesse, en songeant au changement qui va peut-être en résulter pour elles. N'étant pas égoïstes, elles désirent le bonheur de leur Chef avant le leur. Elles n'oublieront jamais les bienfaits dont elles ont été comblées depuis trois ans; son nom restera sur toutes les lèvres, pour dire combien il fut aimé de tout son Personnel.[57]
>
> [The nurses of the Women's Service wish to express their sincere congratulations to their *médecin-chef*. They heard with pleasure of her success in this difficult competitive examination, where she triumphed so easily through her great learning. Their joy is tempered by sadness, however, thinking of the changes that may occur for them. Yet, not wanting to be selfish, they wish for their *chef's* happiness before their own. They will never forget the great benefits they have had from her leadership in the past three years. Her name will remain on all their lips, showing how much she was loved by her staff. [Eleven signatures]]

56 Anon, *The Paris Times*, 325 (1925).

57 Corr.Châlons Nursing Staff & CP, PRFP (1925).

This letter and several sentimental poems from the same source reveal the affection and esteem in which Pascal was held by her staff. For all her impatience with officialdom, Pascal inspired great loyalty among hospital personnel throughout her career – save at Prémontré, where she had clashed with the nuns. She seems to have learned lessons from those conflicts, exercising considerable tact when instituting her *Institut médico-pédagogique*. Significantly too, Pascal's tenure at Châlons coincided with a cessation of pleas to the Ministry, whose beleaguered civil servants could breathe more easily. At Châlons, she had found an arena for action and for her talents, only relinquished for the prize of *médecin-chef* in the Paris region.

7. Moisselles and Maison Blanche, 1925–37

Having succeeded at her second attempt in the *Concours des Asiles de la Seine* in December 1925, Pascal was appointed as medical director of the *Asile de Moisselles*, north of Paris, taking up her appointment in February 1926.[1] As the first woman to pass the highly competitive entry examination to the sought-after posts in the Paris region, she attracted immediate press publicity. The *Paris Times* and *La Française* dedicated articles to her.[2] Like many journalists, the *Times* reporter focused on what he saw as her feminine qualities: 'Her charm, her beauty, her great goodness of heart, as well as her quick intelligence are testified to by all those who work with her.'[3]

Élise Émile-Magne, writing in *La Française*, reads Pascal's career as a prime illustration of feminist efforts first to enter, and then to succeed in, previously all-male professions: 'Son triomphe, après tant de labeur et tant d'obstacles surmontés, restera un exemple dans les annales du féminisme [Her triumph after so much toil and so many obstacles overcome, will stand as an example in the annals of feminism].[4] Émile-Magne reminds her readers that, in forging

1 Moisselles DACP (19 December 1925); Barbier, *VOCP,* 37. Pascal had previously sat the *concours* in 1922, coming fifth out of ten candidates of whom only the top two were admitted. In 1925 she was second out of four candidates. Her results were remarkable:

Service record	9/10
Research and awards	35/40
Clinical oral	17/20
Forensic-medical oral	27/30

2 For the political and social orientation of these newspapers see Claude Bellanger, Jacques Godechot, Pierre Guiral, Fernand Terrou, *Histoire générale de la presse française, II de 1871 à 1940* (Paris: Presses Universitaires de France, 1972), 585.

3 'Woman of the Day', *Paris Times,* PRFP (2 December 1925).

4 Élise Émile-Magne, 'La première femme aliéniste de la Seine' [The first woman psychiatrist in the Seine region] *La Française,* PRFP (1925).

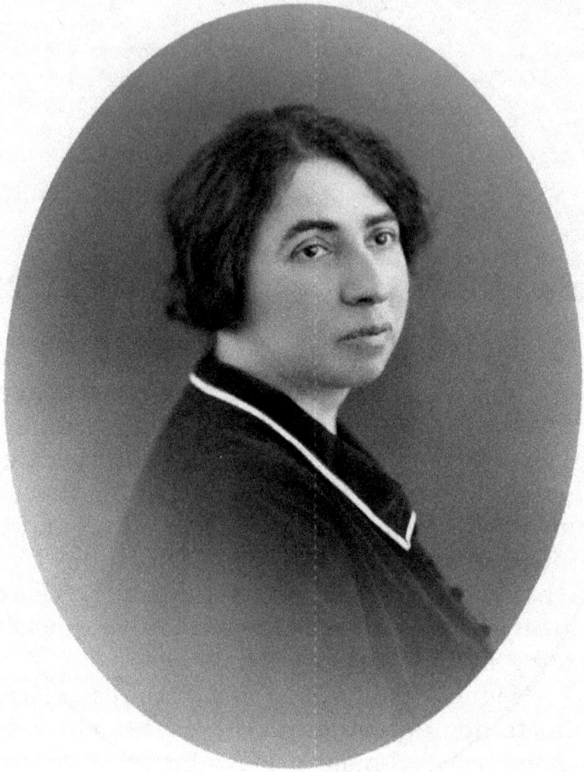

Fig 7. Constance Pascal c. *1926*

her career, Pascal was not without her detractors. From Prémontré, though she was successful in restoring the hospital and dramatically cutting patient death rates, to Châlons sur Marne, where she created the children's school, the reporter describes the opposition she faced from her colleagues as being more daunting than the occasional threat of violence from her deranged patients. It is significant, given Pascal's relatively low profile in suffragist circles, that her feminism is stressed:

> On imagine difficilement, n'est-ce pas? une vie plus laborieusement et plus glorieusement remplie? Mais ce ne fut pas, certes, sans avoir à lutter contre toutes les routines, les préjugés de tous ordres et surtout contre un misonéisme parfois intransigeant. Les femmes de la génération qui monte ne devront pas oublier au prix de quels efforts, de quels sacrifices, de quelles douleurs parfois leurs aînées auront creusé le sillon ('Première Femme aliéniste').

> [It is difficult to imagine, is it not, a life more laboriously and gloriously fulfilled? But this was certainly not without struggling against ingrained routines, all kinds of prejudices and above all a sometimes intransigent misogyny. Young women of the rising generation must not forget what efforts, what sacrifices, what pain sometimes it cost their foremothers to break the path on which they walk.]

Émile-Magne, who must have based her article on an interview with Pascal, accepted, perhaps uncritically, the latter's account of her professional difficulties. While one recognizes the cost of Pascal's struggles throughout her career, her official dossiers demonstrate an impatient, often arrogant and demanding personality, unwilling to compromise and driven nearly to the brink by the frustrations attendant on her work. To see what needed improving in the material and mental welfare of her patients and to feel powerless to act reduced Pascal, as one sees from her correspondence with asylum directors and the Ministry, to emotional near-collapse. Nevertheless, her second and successful attempt at the *concours de la Seine* reflects her ambition to succeed in the hierarchical and competitive psychiatric profession. As a woman in a still predominantly male world, she was determined to achieve equality by demonstrating her intellectual and professional competence. At Moisselles she found the ingrained habits and prejudices if not the misogyny emphasized by Émile-Magne in her article. Though she only served there a year before transferring to Maison Blanche in the eastern Parisian suburb of Neuilly, she displayed her characteristic determination, reforming energy and combativeness, but in the process won herself few friends.

About an hour north of Paris by train, Moisselles was a relatively small asylum of some 500 patients, all women and children. In June 1925 the asylum first took 'uneducable children'; by 1926, when Pascal arrived, these numbered 135.[5] Her workload was heavy. She was responsible both for the women, many of them elderly, and the children, as well as the general hospital administration. Leading on from her pioneering work at Châlons, she attempted to improve the physical and educational provision for handicapped children in the hospital. The official neglect with which they were treated emerged in her report of 1926, which exposed the lack of hygiene in the children's ward, leading to epidemics of whooping cough, mumps and typhoid in which forty-three children and eleven women died.[6] Washing facilities for the children, many of whom were incontinent,

5 Rapport Constance Pascal (Moisselles DACP, 1925).

6 Rapport Constance Pascal (Moisselles DACP, 1926).

were non-existent. Pascal took her young charges to the women's bathing quarters, but even here there was little hot water:

> Je signale quelques défectuosités regrettables dans ce service: l'encombrement et l'hydrothérapie insuffisante, qui facilitent la pullulation et la propagation des germes. Pour plus de 100 enfants gâteux, nous n'avons disposé d'aucune baignoire; l'eau chaude manque partout. Nous avons été obligés d'organiser un service d'hydrothérapie régulier pour les enfants dans celui des bains généraux des femmes (Rapport CP Moiselles DACP 1926).
>
> [I would like to draw your attention to some regrettable defects in this service: over-crowding and insufficient hydrotherapy, which encourage the proliferation and propagation of germs. For more than one hundred incontinent children, we have not a single bath; there is no hot water anywhere. We have been forced to organize a regular hydrotherapy service for the children in the women's general bathing areas.]

More positively, nine children who were treated for hereditary syphilis improved sufficiently to be sent to the Colonie de Vaucluse.[7] However, Pascal's attempts to engage teachers for her young charges were met with indifference and hostility. Barbier describes Pascal's disputes over this issue with the higher administration 'à la suite d'un violent conflit en 1926 avec l'administration' [following a violent conflict with the administration in 1926] (*VOCP*, 38). Administrative intransigence was based on a desire to save money and on the widely held view that only 'educable children' should receive instruction.[8] Furthermore, Pascal's zeal in encouraging and defending nursing staff, a much under-rated, under-trained and under-paid but essential part of the asylum system, angered some in the administration:[9]

> Je suis heureuse de pouvoir signaler le dévouement des infirmières et des surveillantes; elles ont rempli leurs fonctions avec beaucoup de cœur, de patience et de vigilance, et c'est grâce à leurs qualités

7 These colonies were residential centres for children and/or adults with learning difficulties, but they had a darker side, in the sometimes brutal treatment of children for experimental purposes. See Loign Le Sonn, 'Les Déboires d'enquête d'Alfred Binet auprès des enfants des écoles primaires de Paris (1897–1905)' Communication au colloque de Limoges (association Française de Sociologie), 7/8 April 2005.

8 For the treatment of children with learning difficulties, see Jacques Duché Didider, *Histoire de la psychiatrie de l'enfant* (Paris: Presses Universitaires de France, 1990).

9 Jacques Chazaud, 'Introduction', Constance Pascal, *Chagrins d'amour et psychoses* [1935] (Paris: L'Harmattan, 2000), iii.

> exceptionnelles que nous avons pu circonscrire les trois grandes épidémies qui ont régné pendant six mois dans le service des enfants (Rapport CP Moiselles DACP, 1926).
>
> [I am happy to be able to mention the devotion of the nurses and assistants; they have carried out their duties with great warmth, patience and vigilance, and it is thanks to their exceptional qualities that we have been able to hold in check the three serious epidemics that broke out over six months in the children's ward.]

Pascal's recognition of the contribution of her female nursing staff became one of the hallmarks of her annual reports. During her year at Moisselles, two vacancies had arisen in the Paris region, the asylums of Perray Vaucluse and Maison Blanche. Turning down Perray Vaculuse, located in a distant southern suburb of Paris, Pascal successfully applied for the post at Maison Blanche, an all-women psychiatric hospital, to which she was appointed in 1927.[10]

Apart from her conflicts with the administration, one of Pascal's principal motives for leaving Moisselles for a psychiatric hospital closer to Paris must have been to avoid the difficult school commute for her daughter, now studying at the Collège Sévigné in the heart of the city. Jeanne Pascal began her studies there in 1926, remaining until 1933 when she transferred to the *Lycée Henri IV*.[11] Her mother had always refused to send her to boarding school and remained closely involved in her education. Both at Prémontré and Châlons, Jeanne had attended the village school. Living in the asylum grounds, she played with the asylum children. The patients, some of whom worked in the house as domestics, formed part of her wider family. Her mother, fond of animals, kept cats, singing birds, dogs, chickens, ducks, pigeons and rabbits. With the move to Paris and Jeanne now nine or ten years old, this country style of living gave way to more formal schooling. Pascal was determined to ensure that her bright and active young daughter received a rigorous academic education.

The Collège Sévigné, a private college founded in 1880 and located in the heart of the Latin Quarter in the fifth *arrondissement*, was the first girls' school to prepare young women for the baccalaureate. For Pascal, its other attraction was that the great friend of her student years, Mathilde Salomon, an inspirational lay educationist, had been the first headmistress there. Jeanne Pascal blossomed in this academic atmosphere and in the 1933 baccalaureate attained excellent results in philosophy: 'j'ai terminé mes études par un triomphe dans le Bac'

10 Moisselles DACP.

11 IJPR, 19 March 2002.

(JPR, Mémoires, MS, PRFP) [I finished my studies with a triumph in the Bac].

Nevertheless, even after the move from Moisselles to Maison Blanche in Neuilly, the practical difficulties for Jeanne to attend school were daunting. She had to be accompanied on the train or metro by a member of her mother's domestic staff, usually a hospital employee. Matters improved in 1929 when, with the help of General Mengin, her mother purchased a car and hired a chauffeur for the school run. The General often took his daughter to lunch (as her mother thought the school meals were insufficiently nourishing), and at weekends he tutored her in maths and Latin. Thus, although Pascal and Mengin kept their households separate, there was a sense of shared family life. Pascal's acute sense of responsibility for her daughter, her careful oversight of her studies and pleasure in Jeanne's intellectual development coexisted with an almost ferocious attachment to her profession and her patients. At home, as a result, there were few leisure activities; no concerts, theatre or cinema, and few visitors. Reading was a great resource, as was classical music on the radio. Pascal supervised her daughter's homework, helped her with her literature and philosophy essays and imbued her with a love of the maxims of Marcus Aurelius and Pascal's *Pensées*. It was a high-minded training for a child, on the pattern of the French intellectual elite. However, though academically extremely able, Jeanne did have a chink in her scholastic armour, namely her weakness in English. Anxious for her to improve, Pascal hired a language tutor, Edmund Rees, a Welsh student then studying in Paris. He became a frequent guest, part of the family circle and many years later Jeanne's husband.

All was not intellectual hot-housing, however. Pascal wanted her daughter to see something of the world, especially given the fact that they had always lived in or near psychiatric hospitals. Jeanne Pascal remembered summer holidays involving trips abroad, to the seaside, or to the Vosges Mountains. There they would be joined by 'the General', or 'Parrain' [Godfather], though he and Pascal kept separate rooms. Pascal's concern appears to have been to foster her daughter's and Mengin's relationship, while distancing herself from him. Jeanne adored 'cet homme robuste, cette main protectrice que je tiens en marchant. Il est pour moi, à la fois, le Jean Valjean et le colonel, père de Marius, dans *Les Misérables*. Il m'arrive de me désoler de le voir retourner à Paris dans le soir pluvieux' (JPR, Mémoires, MS, PRFP) [this strong man, with his protective hand in mine when we were out walking. For me, he was, at the same time, Jean Valjean and Marius's father the Colonel in *Les Misérables*. Sometimes it would break my

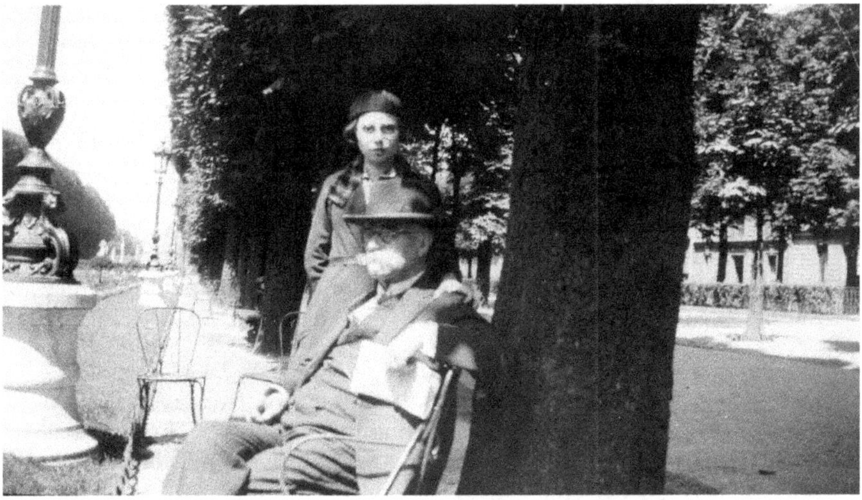

Fig 8. General Mengin and Jeanne Pascal c. *1932*

heart to see him leave on a rainy evening to go home to Paris]. In his later years, Mengin lodged with Baron Reille, a banker and his former chief of staff, a devout Catholic.[12] The Order of St Gregory the Great had been bestowed on Baron Reille by the Vatican in recognition of his loyal support to the Church, but for Jeanne and her mother, aware that the Baron disapproved of Mengin's attachment to his illegitimate daughter, this was additional evidence of his religious bigotry. The General once took his daughter to stay with the Reilles, during her mother's illness (her first bout with cancer and her mastectomy), an experience Jeanne found oppressive. She recalled that the Baron referred to her as 'l'enfant du péché' [the child of sin]. His influence on the General was deeply resented by the Pascals.

Shortly after Jeanne's 14th birthday, on 17 August 1930, Pascal decided to tell her daughter that Mengin was not her godfather but her biological father, a resolution that she had previously communicated to him. In later years Jeanne Pascal Rees recalled the ensuing family drama with some irony:

> Depuis plusieurs semaines, Parrain ne nous a pas rendu visite. On l'attend pour le déjeuner. Ma mère m'emmène dans le petit salon. Chacune assise dans un fauteuil, face à face. Ma mère calmement déclare: 'Il est temps que je te dise que ton Parrain est ton père'. Elle

12 Baron Xavier Reille, 1871–1944: Colonel of Artillery; Commander of the Légion d'Honneur; Croix de guerre 1914–18; Commander of the order of St Gregory the Great; Président of the Compagnie Général Industrielle; Ancien député de la Tarn (1898–1910).

ajoute: 'Il faut deux cellules pour venir au monde. Je suis seule à t'élever; il ne t'a pas reconnue.' La voix s'est entrecoupée, les larmes perlent dans ses yeux. Ces propos sont en grand parti du chinois pour moi. À l'époque, sexe, conception, contrôle de naissance sont des mots tabous. Petit enfant j'avais accepté d'être née dans les choux, puis d'avoir été trouvée, comme notre chien Mimi, dans un caisson de munitions. Une seule donnée solide: que celle que j'appelle ma mère est ma mère; je porte en moi l'empreinte de sa tendresse. Pour le reste, ce 17 août, je suis abasourdi, heureuse que les mains qui me protègent soient celles d'un père, dont les livres de morale de ma petite enfance m'ont décrit les vertus bienfaisantes (JPR, Mémoires, MS, PRFP).

[For several weeks, Godfather had not been to see us. He was expected for lunch. My mother took me into the little salon. We each sat in an armchair, face to face. My mother announced quietly: 'The time has come to tell you that your Godfather is your father.' She added: 'Two cells are necessary to create life. I have brought you up on my own; he has not acknowledged you [*in law*].' Her voice trembled; there were tears in her eyes. Most of this speech was Greek to me. At that time, words like sex, conception, birth control etc. were taboo. As a young child I had accepted that I was born in the cabbage-patch, then that I had been found, like our dog Mimi, in a munitions crate. The only solid fact I knew was that the person I called Mother was my mother; her love was imprinted in me. As far as this new information was concerned, I was stunned, but happy to know that those protective hands belonged to a father, for the moral tales of my childhood had told me all about the benefits and virtues of fathers.]

Edmund Rees, who was invited to this momentous luncheon party, remembered that there seemed to be a great deal of tension in the air. He was not, of course, privy to the secret. Apart from the revelation that 'Parrain' was her father, Jeanne Rees's account contains another intriguing comment: 'The only solid fact I knew was that the person I called Mother was my Mother.' Both in written communications and in conversation she affirmed her maternal heritage and only seems to have discovered that Pascal, her biological mother, had adopted her after her death. For his part, the General wrote to Pascal, of whom he seems to have been in awe, in a formal, rhetorical style:

Je ne veux pas attendre mon retour à Paris pour vous dire combien j'ai été touché de votre attitude vis-à-vis Jeanne. Vous ne m'avez pas caché que le moment semblait imminent où Jeanne, très éveillée, voudrait avoir des détails précis sur son arrivée au monde. Avec un tact parfait et une délicatesse exquise, auxquels je rends hommage, vous luis avez dérobé la vérité, et Jeanne m'a écrit des lettres sublimes débordantes d'affection pour vous, et pleines de reconnaissance pour vos attentions de tous les jours. Je pouvais craindre de sa part, pour des raisons multiples, une froideur significative à mon égard. Grande a été mon émotion, quand elle m'a demandé la permission de m'appeler son petit papa, et de partager avec vous l'affection qu'elle porte à l'auteur de ses jours. Je ne puis que continuer à lui verser une adoration sans bornes, à lui consacrer à tous les instants toutes les forces dont je suis encore capable. (C'est bien peu au regard de ce qu'elle m'a apporté; de la consolation et du bonheur pour mes vieux jours.) Mais guidé par votre affection pour elle, je ne négligerai aucun moyen de prendre une petite part dans les efforts constants que vous ne lui ménagez pas, pour lui faciliter son entrée dans la vie et lui préparer une carrière aussi heureuse que possible (Corr Justin Mengin & CP PRFP, 26 August 1930).

[I do not want to wait until I am back in Paris to say how touched I was by your attitude towards Jeanne. You had not concealed from me that the time seemed imminent when Jeanne, who is such an alert child, would want to know the precise details of her arrival in the world. With perfect tact and an exquisite delicacy, which I cannot praise enough, you unveiled the truth to her and Jeanne has written me some beautiful letters, overflowing with affection for you and full of gratitude for your daily care. For a number of reasons, I was afraid she might behave with significant coldness towards me. How great was my emotion when she asked for permission to call me her 'petit papa', and to share with you the affection she feels for the creator of her being. I can only continue to show her my limitless adoration and to offer her without stint all the strength that still remains to me. (It is little enough compared to what she has given me: consolation and happiness in my old age.) But, guided by your affection for her, I shall not fail, by any means at my disposal, to take some little part in the constant unsparing efforts with which you try to ease her entry into life and prepare for her as happy a future as possible.]

In spite of sentimental flourishes ('how great was my emotion'; 'limitless adoration'), Mengin promises nothing concrete, and indeed sounds a note of vulnerability ('all the strength that still remains to me' and 'consolation and happiness in my old age'). In 1930, Mengin was seventy-four years old and already in failing health. His letter to Jeanne emphasizes sentiment at the expense of any concrete commitment. He recalls that he had once resolved to devote his life to her, surrounding her with paternal care, but scandal mongering by malicious persons had caused him, he says, to see her only occasionally:

Oui, je suis très heureux de te redire ce mot que je brûlais de crier depuis si longtemps. Je me vois encore à Châlons, pleurant d'émotions contenues quand tu me disais un jour en revenant du Collège, oui, mon petit parrain, je t'aime comme si tu étais mon papa. En ce moment j'ai renouvelé le serment de me consacrer entièrement à toi, de ne vivre que pour toi en t'entourant d'une sollicitude paternelle de tous les instants. Et cela à tel point que j'avais formé le projet de ne plus te quitter. [...] Il m'en a coûté de ne plus te voir que par intervalles. [...] Maintenant plus que jamais, je te [donnerai? illegible] ma vive affection, ne cherchant que ton bonheur en tout durant les dernières années qui me restent à vivre (Corr Justin Mengin & Jeanne Pascal, PRFP, 26 August 1930).

[How happy I am to repeat the words I have wanted for so long to say to you. I well remember, at Châlons, weeping with suppressed emotion when you came back from school one day and said: 'Yes, dear Godfather, I love you as if you were my own daddy'. I vowed at that moment to dedicate myself completely to you, to live for you, surrounding you every minute with fatherly care. I swore I would never leave you. It pained me to see you so rarely [...] Now more than ever, I offer you my deep affection, seeking your happiness in everything for the last few years that remain to me.]

What is particularly revealing in his letters is the fear of gossip about Jeanne's origins that obsessed both parents and the pressure of public opinion, whether real or imagined, on them. Although Mengin says he rejoices in Jeanne's new knowledge, he did not sign his letter, presumably so that it could not be used as documentary evidence in a paternity suit, or as promising legal recognition. Furthermore, in Pascal's eyes, Mengin's epistolary effusions were suspect: 'Ces sentiments sont faux; c'est de l'attendrissement passager' [These expressions of feeling are false. It's just the emotion of the moment].[13]

For Jeanne's part, while nothing was said explicitly, she knew she must keep her parentage secret. Having been given the minimum of information by her mother, who seems to have conveyed a largely unintelligible explanation of the sexual act, while precluding, with her customary authority and hauteur, any further discussion, it was made perfectly clear to the young girl that there were to be no further revelations about her parents' love affair, nor must she ever reveal the information to which she had just been made privy:

Superficiellement, notre routine n'a pas changée et j'ai continué à l'appeler Parrain. Simplement, j'étais dépositaire du secret qui bouillonnait en moi. Ma mère a connu de tristes moments. Son enfant semblait l'abandonner pour aller dans les bras du père qui d'après elle aurait pu me reconnaître. À ce moment sa générosité a été admirable.

13 Pencilled note by CP to Jeanne Pascal on letter of JM to JP (PRFP, 26 August 1930).

> Elle a tout fait pour faciliter cet amour filial qui ne lui était pas destiné (JPR, Mémoires, MS, PRFP).

> [On the surface nothing in our routine changed and I went on calling him 'Godfather'. At the same time I had been given a secret to keep that seethed within me. My mother was often unhappy. It was as if her child was abandoning her in favour of the father who, she felt, could have given me legal recognition. Her generosity at that time was truly admirable. She did everything to encourage this filial love which was not directed towards her.]

Had Mengin given his daughter legal recognition, Jeanne would still have been illegitimate but she would have gained inheritance rights on the paternal side. However, Pascal's anger and desire for him to recognize Jeanne were more to do with giving her daughter the father's name, public acknowledgement of his paternal responsibility and a civil identity through the father.

With the move to Maison Blanche in 1927, Pascal and Jeanne were lodged in a comfortable house with a garden near the hospital gates, where the family's four dogs and seven cats could be accommodated. The hospital, opened in 1900, was built to a similar pattern to other Parisian asylums, consisting of large wards, joined by covered walkways.[14] At this period it was exclusively for women, divided into 'sections' or departments. Pascal was in charge of the First Section, which eventually in 1934 moved to new premises, becoming the Third Section.[15] The three principal sources of Pascal's clinical – as opposed to research – activity for this period are found, firstly, in her annual official report to the Departmental Prefect; secondly, in her Maison Blanche dossier; and thirdly in a series of interviews and tours of the asylum that she gave to three reporters from popular journals in 1932 and 1933. Her annual reports and her personal dossier are revealing about asylum conditions and her efforts to improve them.[16]

A hospital psychiatrist was responsible for the medical as well as the mental state of her/his patients. In the annual reports, psychiatric and medical conditions appear inextricably mixed. In 1929, for example,

14 Barbier, *VOCP*, 38–39; *1900–2000: Maison Blanche: le centenaire, actes de la journée du centenaire de Maison Blanche, 22 juin 2000*, ed. by Michel Caire and others (EPS, 2001), 37–43.

15 Pascal was officially installed as *médecin-chef* of the first section on 1 February 1927 (Procès-Verbal de l'Installation de Mademoiselle Pascal, nommée Médecin-Chef de Service à l'asile de Maison-Blanche, Préfecture du Département de la Seine, Maison Blanche, DACP).

16 I am most grateful to Dr Michel Caire for access to Pascal's personal dossier at Maison Blanche.

Pascal's report for her department sets out the number of patients treated in the year (690) and the numbers remaining after transfer, improvement, cure or decease (478). Diagnostic categories of patients' illnesses follow: general paralysis (syphilis), 18; persecution delirium, 29; *dementia praecox*, 22; manic depressive psychosis, 27; deceased, 49. After the mandatory statistical section, Pascal summarized the year's major challenges: treatment of syphilitic patients, control of tuberculosis and treatment of a dysentery outbreak, as well as her recommendations for improved therapies via the introduction of a laboratory to assist research in biology, radiology and bacteriology for mental illnesses.[17] As was clear from these reports, physical illnesses, many of them preventable, afflicted significant numbers of patients. Every year tuberculosis killed six to eight patients until it was controlled in 1932. Overcrowding remained a central concern. In 1929, for example the number of patients treated by Pascal was 690, yet by 1932 it had risen to 811. In the asylum as a whole, from 1909 to 1934, the population almost doubled from 1200 to 2258.[18] Living conditions were spartan and since many patients were incontinent, hygiene – or the lack of it – was a major concern.

From 1930 to 1936 Pascal and her colleagues wrote repeatedly to the director complaining of overcrowding. On 29 November 1930 they sent the director a detailed request for additional beds and nursing staff, pointing out that many of the new patients transferred from Sainte-Anne, where they had been assessed, were highly agitated, violent and in need of close supervision, which present staffing resources could not provide.[19] Three months later, on 14 February 1931, Pascal wrote again, detailing her concerns about overcrowding, in a vivid picture of life for her patients:

> J'ai l'honneur de vous informer qu'en l'état actuel de l'organisation de mon service, il ne m'est pas possible de tenir ma promesse: accepter soixante malades en plus de mon effectif habituel (480 aliénés). Lorsque la Commission spéciale de l'encombrement était venue visiter mon service, il était bien entendu que je devais affecter un dortoir au traitement des nouvelles malades. Pour réaliser cette organisation nouvelle, on m'a promis le personnel nécessaire sans lequel on ne peut assurer aucun traitement, aucune surveillance. Or, rien n'a été fait jusqu'ici. J'ai reçu trente-deux malades au surnombre. J'ai actuellement 512 aliénés. Ces malades occupent le milieu des

17 Rapport Constance Pascal (MBDACP, 1929), 156.

18 Marie-Josèe Moll and Jean-Claude Pèna, 'L'architecture asilaire, de 1900 à nos jours', *Maison Blanche le centenaire*, 37–43.

19 Constance Pascal and two others (signatures illegible), to Director (MBDACP, 29 November 1930).

dortoirs, les interstices des lits placés sur les côtés, même dans les services des grandes agitées. L'encombrement atteint déjà son point maximum.

De plus: une épidémie de grippe (35 malades) règne dans mon service. Elle a été provoquée par une entrante qui est venue de Staint-Anne avec 40° de température.

Il me semble qu'il y a lieu de prendre des mesures urgentes au point de vue de l'encombrement actuel. J'ai toujours le plus vif désir d'être utile à l'Administration du service des aliénés pour parer à la crise actuelle, mais j'estime qu'il s'agit là d'un devoir supérieur: *l'intérêt des malades*. Nous ne pouvons plus les soigner. Le personnel ne suffit plus à la surveillance. Comme mon collègue, le Dr Demay, je demande la limitation de l'encombrement actuel faute de nouvelle organisation. Je demande que la Commission de l'encombrement vienne constater elle-même l'impossibilité de dépasser ce chiffre (510 malades) et les résultats d'un encombrement devenu dangereux et nuisible (Maison Blanche DACP 14 February 1931).

[I write to inform you that in the present state of organization in my department, it is impossible for me to fulfil my promise to accept sixty patients in addition to my normal allocation (480). When the Special Commission on Overcrowding visited my department, I agreed to their request that I allocate one ward for the use of new patients. In order to achieve this, I was promised the staff needed to ensure the necessary treatment and supervision. Up to now, nothing has been done. I have taken in thirty-two patients above the maximum: I now have 512. These patients are occupying the middle of the wards and the spaces between the beds at both sides, even in the wards with the most disturbed patients. Overcrowding has already reached its absolute maximum.

In addition we have a 'flu epidemic at the moment (thirty-five cases). It was brought in by a patient who arrived from Sainte Anne with a temperature of 40°. In the light of this overcrowding I believe we need urgent action. I am fully committed to helping the Administration of the Service for the Insane in the present crisis, but I believe there is a higher priority here: *the needs of the patients*. We can no longer care for them. We no longer have enough staff to supervise them. Along with my colleague Dr Demay, I ask you to put an end to this overcrowding, unless we are able to reorganize the service. I would like ask the Commission for Overcrowding to come and see for itself the impossibility of raising numbers above 510, and the effects of this overcrowding, which is fast becoming dangerous and harmful.]

The situation had not improved by the following year. Pascal protested to the Director that her department was still carrying an impossible load:

L'encombrement d'un service n'est pas seulement fonction de locaux, mais encore de toutes les autres possibilités médicales. Je n'ai qu'un seul interne pour assurer les soins à 526 malades. Je ne comprends pas pourquoi on impose constamment à mes collaborateurs et à moi un surcroît de travail. On ne tient pas compte des soins à donner à 89 malades de plus, aux écritures à faire, du Parloir qui est devenu une vraie foire, de l'impossibilité de baigner toutes les malades agitées et anxieuses. [...] Je vous prie de vouloir bien signaler à Mr le Préfet, le danger qu'il y a d'augmenter le chiffre des malades dans mon service. Il a été organisé pour recevoir 375 malades, il contient actuellement 526 malades. Il a fourni tous les efforts. Il ne peut plus supporter une nouvelle surcharge (CP to Director, MBDACP, 4 February 1932).

[Overcrowding in a department is not just a matter of space – it affects all the other aspects of medical care. I have only one intern for 526 patients. I do not understand why extra work is constantly imposed on my colleagues and me. No one seems to take into account what it means to care for 89 more patients, the additional paperwork, pandemonium in the common-room, trying to bath all these disturbed and anxious women. [...] I ask you, please, to alert the Prefect to the dangers of increasing the number of patients in my department. It was set up to take 375 patients and it now has 526. We have done everything asked of us. We simply cannot manage any more.]

In spite of Pascal's protestations, numbers continued to creep upwards. From the 526 patients that she considered intolerable in 1932, the number rose to 564 and would reach 575. A letter of 1 April 1934 conveys her increased irritation, concluding:

Je répète: mon service a fourni tous les efforts; les dortoirs sont encombrés, les couloirs exigus surchargés de matelas par terre, les salles de réunion sont devenues étouffantes. Après une longue expérience de l'encombrement, je puis dire que le service ne pourra plus supporter beaucoup de malades. Il me faudra utiliser les réfectoires. Il faut mettre les malades là où il y a de la place, et non là où il n'y en a plus, où les efforts sont épuisés. Non pour me permettre de ne rien faire, mais, par humanité pour les malades couchées par terre et qui étouffent, sans air respirable.[20]

[I repeat: my department has made every effort demanded of it; the wards are full to bursting, the cramped corridors piled with mattresses on the floor, the common rooms are stifling. After years of such overcrowding, it is clear to me that this department cannot manage so many patients. I will end up having to use the dining-halls. We should put patients where there is some room, not where there is none, where all efforts have been exhausted. I'm not trying to

20 Corr CP & Dir (MBDACP, 1 April 1934).

> save myself work, it's a question of pure humanity. These patients are suffocating, sleeping on the floor where the air is barely breathable.]

She ends with an angry coda: 'Mais l'incident est clos pour moi. Je ne puis continuer aucune discussion; je sais maintenant que j'aurai toujours tort, malgré l'évidence des faits et ma protestation justifiée' [But, as far as I'm concerned, the matter is closed. I cannot go on discussing it; I know now that I will always be in the wrong, in spite of the factual evidence and my justified protests]. Her relations with the Director, who was probably trammelled by budgetary constraints and unable or unwilling to change the situation, had clearly deteriorated badly.

Conditions for the nursing staff were still very poor (there was little privacy for those obliged to live in the dormitories) and they were often, particularly at night, exposed to attack from the more violent patients. Pascal's 1932 report to the inspectors emphasizes the risks overcrowding posed for her staff as well as for the patients:

> Je me permets de me plaindre de cet encombrement, non pour moi, mais pour les malades qui vivent pêle-mêle et pour le personnel qui ne peut plus assurer une surveillance stricte. Les malades dangereuses vivent côte à côte avec les malades inoffensives. Le service de veille, le plus pénible, continue à être assuré par une seule veilleuse dans le service dit de 'tranquilles'. En cas de menace de la part d'une aliénée devenue subitement dangereuse, elle est exposée à la mort; elle ne pourra même pas appeler au secours, étant seule, la nuit, dans un pavillon de 85 malades! J'ai signalé le fait à plusieurs reprises; il me *paraît d'une importance majeure.*[21]

> [I feel I must make a complaint about this overcrowding, not for myself but for the patients, who live together cheek by jowl, and for the staff, who can no longer maintain adequate supervision. Dangerous patients are accommodated alongside harmless ones. Night duty, which is the most difficult, is still carried out by a single member of staff assigned to oversee the so-called calm patients. In the event of threats from a lunatic who has suddenly become dangerous, she is in danger of her life; she cannot even call for help, being alone at night in a ward with 85 patients! I have reported this danger several times; it seems to me of *paramount importance.*]

Her representations to the Director resulted in a move to a new Third Section in 1934, with a reduced total of 400 patients. Pascal rejoiced in the improved conditions for staff and patients, for the new Section offered a genuine hospital service for both physical

21 Rapport Constance Pascal (MBDACP, 1932), 174.

and mental illnesses – bright, cheerful, airy and well-heated wards, washable floors, bathing facilities, good furniture and individual wardrobes for the patients' belongings.[22] The enumeration of these improvements serves to demonstrate the deplorable state of facilities prior to the move. In that year, Pascal goes on to say, the effect on the patients' general health was striking: a 'flu epidemic which was raging elsewhere spared her ward. Nonetheless, conditions at Maison Blanche continued to be difficult, as an attack on a nurse in 1936 demonstrates.

On 21 February Pascal wrote a terse note to the Director. Her predictions on the dangers of staff shortages coupled with overcrowding had unfortunately proved correct:

> Je vous informe que ce matin à 7 heures, il y a eu un incident grave dans mon service, au 6me pavillon. L'infirmière Madame Besse distribuait le pain aux malades de son dortoir et sans qu'elle s'y attende, elle fût assaillie brutalement par derrière par la malade Carron. Prise aux cheveux et serrée à la gorge, elle put appeler au secours. Heureusement, la surveillante Mme Nourrisson, se trouvait dans son bureau et elle put la secourir. J'attire votre attention sur ce fait grave qui est dû à l'encombrement et à l'insuffisance croissante du personnel. Le 6me pavillon ne devait recevoir que 42 malades agitées et dangereuses et nous en avons 53 (MBDACP, 21 February 1936).

> [This is to inform you that this morning at 7 o'clock there was a serious incident in my department, on the 6th ward. The nurse, Mme Besse, was giving out bread to the patients in her dormitory when, without warning, she was violently attacked from behind by the patient Carron. Though she had been grabbed by her hair and was being held by the throat, she managed to call for help. Luckily, the supervisor, Mme Nourrisson, was in her office and was able to come to her aid. I draw your attention to this serious incident which is due to overcrowding and the ever-increasing shortage of staff. The 6th ward is meant to hold 42 disturbed and dangerous patients and we currently have 53.]

The nurse's narrow escape forced the Director, who had repeatedly complained to his superiors at the Prefecture of the effects of overcrowding, to write forcefully on 26 February 1936 to the Director of Departmental Affairs:

> J'ai l'honneur de vous transmettre le rapport ci-joint de Mlle le Dr Pascal, relatif à un incident qui aurait pu avoir de graves conséquences. À plusieurs reprises je vous ai fait part des inconvénients multiples d'une surpopulation excessive et de l'arrivée quasi-journalière de

22 Rapport Constance Pascal (MBDACP, 1934), 87.

nouvelles malades. Je sais que cet état de choses n'est pas particulier à Maison-Blanche et je ne méconnais pas non plus l'impérieuse nécessité d'hospitaliser les malades admises à Ste-Anne. Toutefois, je crois devoir vous signaler à nouveau une situation qui s'aggrave de jour en jour, en attirant votre attention sur les dangers qui peuvent en résulter.

La population aliénée atteint aujourd'hui 2,692. L'état sanitaire est déplorable par suite de l'épidémie de grippe qui sévit aussi bien chez les malades que parmi le personnel. On relève les chiffres de 40 malades grippées alitées et 15 à 18 infirmières indisponibles pour maladie par section. D'autre part, il ne suffit pas seulement de caser les malades tant bien que mal sur des matelas entre les lits ou dans les salles de réunion, il faut encore les nourrir, les vêtir et les blanchir. Or, depuis longtemps et avant même qu'il y ait encombrement, la nécessité d'agrandir les services généraux avait été reconnue. L'extension des locaux à usage de buanderie, lingerie, cuisine, a été décidée et les travaux viennent de commencer obligeant à des installations de fortune, ce qui n'est pas pour faciliter la marche des services les plus importants. C'est conscient de ma responsabilité et de celle de mes collaborateurs que je demande que les convois soient suspendus tout au moins jusqu'à ce que de nouvelles places deviennent disponibles (MBDACP, 26 February 1936).

[I enclose a report from Dr Pascal relative to an incident which could have had serious consequences. I have informed you many times already of the many problems arising from an excessive over-population and the almost daily arrival of new patients. I know this state of affairs is not unique to Maison Blanche and I am not unaware of the urgent necessity of finding hospital places for patients admitted to Sainte-Anne. Nevertheless, I must again draw your attention to this situation, which is getting worse by the day, and the dangers that may result.

The population of mental patients has today reached the total of 2,692. Sanitary facilities are deplorable, following the 'flu epidemic which ravaged the patients as well as the staff. We had 40 patients in bed with 'flu and 15 to 18 nurses in each department unavailable for work. Moreover, it is not enough to squeeze the patients in as best we can on mattresses between the beds or in the common rooms; they also need food, clothing and laundry. Indeed, for some time now, even before we were overcrowded, the need to improve the general services has been recognized. Extensions to the laundry, sewing room and kitchen were agreed and the works had just started, necessitating makeshift arrangements which in themselves made it difficult to carry out the most essential services. Conscious of my responsibilities and those of my colleagues, I ask you to suspend any further transfer of patients until at least new places become available.]

The Director's letter details the same complaints that Pascal had been making over the preceding six years, with the addition that efforts to improve 'general services' had resulted in disruption in the wards. With the likely prospect of staff or patients in his charge being seriously injured or killed, he demanded, as she had long done, a halt to admissions until resources were significantly increased. Her representations had proved to be fully justified, though it required a near tragedy to validate them.

The other leverage that Pascal employed to effect change was to publicize the sufferings of mentally ill patients and to open the secretive world of mental hospitals to the public. She had recourse to the popular, as opposed to the academic, psychiatric press, in three extensive interviews she gave to journalists Louis Roubaud, Paul Allard and Georges Ricou in 1932–33. While recognizing that she wished to show the public something of the tormented lives of seriously mentally ill patients, one is nevertheless struck by the potentially exploitative nature of her material. There was no question of patients having given, or indeed being capable of giving, their consent to appearing in this journalistic gallery of madness, though their full names were withheld.

Roubaud's articles appeared in *Détective*, a magazine specialising in *faits divers*.[23] *Détective* boasted talented writers like Georges Simenon and Roubaud himself, who was a leading investigative journalist. He had attracted publicity by his investigation of children's reform schools which he termed penal colonies, publishing in 1925, *Les Enfants de Caïn*.[24] That Pascal had access to these writers demonstrates the breadth of her acquaintance within the Parisian circles of the Left. Roubaud's report, in deference to his magazine's title, reads like a crime novel where the crime is the murder of the souls of the young women patients interviewed, Pascal is the chief detective and he her Watson.[25] Roubaud was intrigued by Pascal's efforts to unlock her patients' stories by recourse to forms of chemical shock therapy, employing the technique in order to free the patient's memory of precipitating trauma. The patients featured in his exposé were in advanced stages of psychosis, often incapable of speech, sexually disinhibited, or locked in infantile regression. The chemical

23 Christophe Charle, *Le Siècle de la presse* (Paris: Seuil, 2004), 331–34. *Faits divers* are short news items, often concerning criminal or sensational events.

24 Anne Boissel "Les enfants de Caïn, Louis Roubaud", *La lettre de l'enfance et de l'adolescence* 1/2006 (no. 63), pp. 7–10, www.cairn.info/revue-lettre-de-l-enfance-et-de-l-adolescence-2006-1-page-7.htm [accessed 19 September 2012].

25 Louis Roubaud, 'Démons et déments', *Détective* (December, 1932).

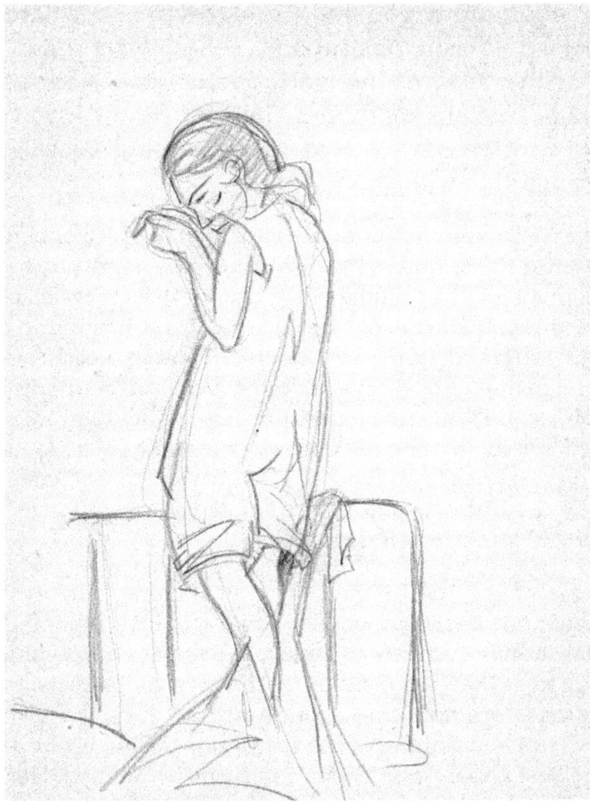

Fig 9. Patient at Maison Blanche, artist unknown

experiments to which Pascal subjected her patients were designed to make possible an approximation of Freud's talking cure. Roubaud's account of this process is frankly *romanesque,* partly for the sake of local colour but principally to convey the horror of each patient's journey into madness. He describes Pascal as the learned interpreter of their stories: 'Le plus subtil, le plus ardent, le plus doux des détectives. [...] sans chimie ni scalpel, la savante demoiselle analyse et dissèque' ('Démons', 5) [the most subtle, passionate and gentle of detectives. [...] With neither drugs nor scalpel, the learned lady analyses and dissects].

The second exposé, Paul Allard's 'Folles d'amour' [Mad with/ for love] appeared in *Vu,* a picture magazine featuring a wide range of contentious topics on social, moral and political issues, the arts, entertainment and anything outré or sensational. With its lavish illustrations, *Vu* was at the forefront of photographic journalism, employing photomontage and rotogravure.[26] Allard's article, accompanied by lavish illustrations, follows a similar pattern to Roubaud's, with a tour of the wards, interviews with patients and explanations of Pascal's methods. The sorrows of love from which these patients suffer, says Allard, paraphrasing Pascal, signify far more than romantic melancholy:

> Le chagrin de l'amour est la douleur de ce qui n'est plus, et l'effort de renaissance de ce qu'on voudrait être. Le chagrin d'amour n'est plus seulement un état d'âme triste, inquiet où révolté. Il devient une peine organique, un mal physique qui perturbe gravement le sentiment vital. [...] Il y a des choses qu'on n'ose pas écrire: imaginez-vous ce que peut être le spectacle donné à chaque heure du jour, par les scatophiles. En voici une – c'est une jeune fille du grande monde. Elle se tord sur son lit. Ses yeux sont hagards. Le cri de la Jungle? Le voici! Nous touchons là au fond de l'instinct libéré, déchaîné. Le plus élémentaire des instincts humains; celui de l'alimentation est perverti d'une manière affreuse et indicible.[27]
>
> [The sorrow of love is the pain of what is gone, and the effort to recreate what one desires to be. The sorrow of love is not only a state of spiritual sadness, anxiety or revolt. It becomes an organic grief, a physical distress that seriously disturbs the vital instincts. [...] There are things one dare not write about: imagine the sight, visible at all hours of the day and night, of the scatophiles. Here is one – a young lady of the best society. She twists and turns on her bed. Her eyes are wild. She shrieks like a jungle animal. We are touching the lowest depths of unleashed, untamed instincts. Here, the most elementary of human instincts, that of nourishment, is being perverted, in a dreadful and unspeakable way.]

Allard couples his pleasurable frisson of horror at the scenes of mental disequilibrium he has witnessed with admiration for Pascal's calm, expertise and compassion.

Georges Ricou, reporting for *Le Petit Journal*, devotes three columns and a photograph to Pascal. Consistent with the popular and populist editorial stance of the paper,[28] the article begins with an appraisal of Pascal's work in terms of gender stereotypes. She incarnates the maternal ethos: 'Femme, la Doctoresse Pascal a la sensibilité, l'intuition, instinctive et cultivée, l'élan généreux de tendresse et d'amour qui appartiennent naturellement à la femme' [A true

26 Michel Frizot, 'Looking at Vu: a photographic magazine, 1928–1940', www.mep-fr.org/us/actu/vu.htm [accessed 19 September 2012].

27 Paul Allard, 'Folles d'amour', *Vu* (PRFP, 1933), 1143–44.

28 Charle, 2004, 102–106.

woman, Dr Pascal has the sensitivity, the intuition, both innate and learned, and the generous impulse of tenderness and love that belong naturally to the fair sex].[29] He also recognizes her as an innovator, whose example would attract young women to join the psychiatric profession. For her part Pascal is quoted as saying that psychiatry as a profession is especially well suited to women, perhaps co-opting a gender stereotype for feminist ends. The numbers of women in psychiatry, it should be noted, were still not overwhelming by 1933: only six alongside 121 men.[30] Ricou gives due weight to Pascal's scientific credentials and to her wide humanist culture. But he reads Pascal's devotion to her patients as an example of women's natural capacity for self-sacrifice, an assumption that virtually negates any willpower or moral credit for her actions:

> Je vois bien la doctoresse Pascal parmi ses malades. Je vois surtout une femme au grand cœur parmi d'autres femmes qui souffrent et sont misérables. Deux destins d'humanité qui s'unissent dans une œuvre salvatrice: une femme de science et de pitié qui se penche et s'efforce de tirer d'autres femmes hors du gouffre infernal de folie (Ricou, 'Les Cloîtres', 3).

> [I still can see Dr Pascal surrounded by her patients. I see above all a kind-hearted woman among other women who are suffering and deprived. Two human destinies come together in this work of succour; a woman of science bends down, moved by pity, to help other women up out of the infernal abyss of madness.]

Pascal was indeed devoted to her patients, as is evidenced by both her published works and her private correspondence. For Ricou this admirable devotion could be represented as a new aspect of women's traditional destiny. From the perspective of popular journalism, a woman psychiatrist was less a threatening 'new woman' than a traditional feminine archetype of the carer.

Nonetheless, it is evident that the three reporters who, on their separate visits, followed Pascal round the wards with some trepidation, and who reflected popular fears and fascination provoked by the closed world of the asylums, also marvelled at her courage and professional composure. Though compassionate towards her patients, as the reporters noted, she was not sentimental about them. Her daughter remembered 'manufactured' rages when patients lost

29 Georges Ricou, 'Dans les cloîtres de la folie: la Doctoresse Pascal', *Le Petit Journal* (1 January 1933).

30 Liste des membres, Société Médico-Psychologique, *Annales médico-psychologiques* (January 1936). I am indebted to Dr Michel Caire for this reference.

control of themselves, a tactic to jolt them back to better behaviour.[31] In her psychiatric persona, she maintained a necessary detachment, whilst never forgetting the mental torments of the wounded beings she was dealing with. Her letters to the Maison Blanche Director protesting at living conditions for patients also demonstrate the extent to which she felt the indignity and degradation of the conditions in which many of them were forced to live.

From the professional activity recorded in the years 1927–37, one would have no idea of the cancer that struck Pascal in 1928, for which she underwent a mastectomy. Awaiting the results of her biopsy, she wrote to the General: 'Je ne peux pas vous exprimer mon angoisse. Dès que j'aurai les résultats je vous enverrai un télégramme. Merci de tout ce que vous faites pour ma petite' (Corr CP & JM PRFP 1928) [I can't tell you how anxious I am. As soon as I have the results I will send you a telegram. Thank you for everything you are doing for my little girl] – not, one notes, 'our little girl'. Mengin took Jeanne to stay with the Baron Reille and his wife during Pascal's convalescence. Thereafter she lived under the shadow of potential recurrence, hiding her fears from Jeanne until 1937, when the illness reasserted itself.[32] The likely prospect of an early death explains many of Pascal's anxieties about Jeanne's future – her hope that Mengin would give his daughter legal recognition, her insistence that she excel in her studies, and her decision in 1934 to buy a house in the Marne Valley in the village of Chantemanche, which became her material legacy to her daughter.

In 1932, the General, who had long been ailing, died at the Val de Grâce Military Hospital and was buried with full military honours. For reasons of discretion, Pascal did not visit him during his last illness, but sent him his favourite dishes, which she had prepared herself. Jeanne went daily, as the hospital was close to the Collège Sévigné:

> Il m'arrivait de croiser dans les couloirs de l'hôpital les belles Mesdames de la haute société aristocratique et militaire qui exaltaient le mourant. Il était remarquable. Il a fait carrière malgré ses petites origines (il était fils d'instituteur). Le jour de l'enterrement dans la belle église du Val de Grâce, en présence du Ministre de la Guerre, nous avons été, ma mère et moi, dans la foule massée à l'entrée sans que le baron Reille fasse un geste pour nous. De quoi haïr le monde catholique et militaire si arrogant (JPR, Mémoires, MS, PRFP).

31 Detail gleaned from personal communication with Mme Rees.

32 IJPR, 19 March 2002.

> [Sometimes, in the hospital corridors, I would cross paths with fine ladies from military or aristocratic high society, singing the praises of the dying man. How remarkable he was, rising so high from such humble origins (he was the son of a primary-school master). The day of the funeral at the grand Val de Grâce Church, in the presence of the Minister of War, my mother and I were among the crowd gathered at the door; the Baron Reille made no sign of acknowledgement to us. Enough to make one hate that arrogant military and Catholic world.]

Pascal's invisibility in this military setting, her status as a non-person at a very public funeral, sums up the dilemmas she had faced with regard to Mengin. Her daughter believed that her mother had loved him during the war years but could not forgive him for not acknowledging either their relationship or his daughter, though he figured as a guardian in Jeanne's adoption papers. For his part, Mengin admired Pascal enormously, kept lists of the articles she had written, was tireless in attempting to promote her career through official channels (as we saw in Chapter IV), ran errands for her in Paris, supervised her investments and was in his own way devoted to her and their daughter, but not to the extent, as we have seen, of granting Jeanne legal recognition: 'Il était le prisonnier de sa famille modeste, fier de lui et fort catholique, prisonnier aussi du milieu social dans lequel il s'était hissé dans sa carrière (JPR, Mémoires, MS, PRFP) [He was the prisoner of his humble origins – his family were proud of him and very Catholic – and also of the social milieu into which had hauled himself in the course of his career].

Mengin gave significant financial support to his daughter during his life, so much so that, in his will, he was obliged to apologize to his two nephews, his legatees, for having nothing to leave them, saying he had suffered stock market losses: 'Les valeurs en portefeuille que je possédais ont servi en majeure partie à soulager les difficultés de la vie, à entretenir ma femme à l'asile d'Evreux et à subvenir à ses charges personnelles' [My stock certificates were largely used to assuage life's difficulties, to support my wife at the Evreux Asylum and subsidize her personal needs].[33] Mengin devotes a paragraph in his will to his religious beliefs: having formerly practised what he calls 'la religion naturelle' [natural religion], he reveals that he had now returned to the Catholic Church. He expresses his gratitude to Colonel Reille, who was doubtless largely responsible for his religious conversion, for welcoming him to his home with so much kindness and disinterestedness. His will makes no reference to Jeanne Pascal, unless the phrase 'life's difficulties' was code for his paternal

33 Justin Mengin, 'Ceci est Mon Testament' (PRFP 1 February 1932).

responsibility. Both parents guarded the secret of Jeanne's parentage until their deaths. Finally, Mme Mengin, long kept as a private patient by her husband in the Evreux Asylum, was discharged the following year, probably because the fees to maintain her had ceased to be paid. When she heard the news, Pascal remarked bitterly to Jeanne that it was too late.[34] Mme Mengin's mental condition on her release and her means of subsistence thereafter remain unknown.

Jeanne Pascal Rees loved and admired both her parents and, drawing, it would appear, on her training as an historian, appreciated them in the context of their socio-historical moment. She understood her mother's anger against Mengin and nevertheless adored her father, whose ebullient and assertive temperament she seems to have inherited. Pascal's judgement of Mengin was stark. She wrote to Jeanne: 'Il n'a pas voulu faire son devoir envers toi. Il en avait les possibilités. Paix à ses cendres, mais trêve aussi aux mensonges' [He chose not to do his duty towards you. He could have done so. Peace to his ashes, but it's time to call a halt to the lies].[35] Jeanne Rees's remembered anger at the 'Catholic and military' society in which her father had lived, reveals much about her and her mother's political and religious orientation. Holding broadly left-wing sympathies, Pascal shared the anti-clericalism of much of her generation of professionals (teachers, civil servants, doctors and lawyers) in the Third Republic. At Prémontré she had encountered hostility from the Catholic nursing sisters and in her psychiatric practice supported the principle of non-religious nursing and teaching staff for her handicapped children. Nevertheless, born into the Eastern Orthodox Church, which she had abandoned, she seems to have felt deep guilt for having given birth to an illegitimate child, a sense of sin without the consolations of religion.[36] Given Pascal's agnosticism, this judgement by Mme Rees might seem excessive, but there is evidence to bear it out. Pascal removed all passages in her War Diary relating to Mengin apart from some early conversations about military strategy; she cut out and destroyed her copy of the lovely photograph of herself as a young woman in *La Vie Heureuse*; she destroyed her correspondence with Mengin and with Jeanne Streicher insofar as it related to Jeanne; she avoided being photographed with Jeanne lest a resemblance be noticed and for many years, she cut off relations with her Romanian family. There is no doubt that she adored her daughter and was

34 IJPR 19 March 2002.

35 CP to JP, note attached to two letters of 26 August 1930 from General Justin Mengin, PRFP.

36 Jeanne Pascal Rees, 'Maladie et mort de C.P, juin/dec. 37', MS (PRFP 2003).

consumed by fears that Jeanne's future would be blighted by her illegitimacy. Her maternity constituted one of the great joys of her life.

Jeanne Streicher, Pascal's most constant friend, a distinguished scholar of seventeenth-century literature and one of the first women to become *agrégée en lettres*, remained loyal to Pascal and Jeanne, whilst disapproving of Pascal's 'faute' [lapse], as she termed it.[37] As we know, Streicher had been appointed Jeanne's guardian in 1924 on her adoption, with Mengin as joint guardian. Her ethical concerns and republican principles paralleled Pascal's own. As Jeanne Pascal Rees recalled:

> À la passion pour les choses de l'esprit qui lui avait fait négliger les simples joies féminines, elle joignait un inébranlable attachement à l'idéal moral qui dirigea toute sa vie. Elle l'avait trouvé dans son éducation républicaine et elle l'enrichissait par la lecture des grands philosophes. Descartes et Kant surtout. Raison, Devoir, Patrie en étaient les piliers; la raison Cartésienne, source de vérité; le devoir Kantien conçu comme un impératif catégorique, jailli de la conscience universelle, l'amour de la patrie, tel que l'enseignaient les républicains après la défaite de 1870 et qui touchait profondément nos filles alsaciennes. Rien d'étroit dans son idéal. Elle portait sur les gens et l'œuvre d'art un regard toujours curieux, tant elle était avide de connaître le vrai et le beau, au-delà des apparences. Il y avait aussi en elle un mélange de puritanisme et de générosité que je n'ai trouvé nulle part ailleurs.[38]
>
> [She had a passion for the life of the mind, which caused her to neglect simple feminine pleasures, and an unwavering attachment to the moral ideal that shaped her whole life. This had its source in her republican education and she enriched it by reading the great philosophers, especially Descartes and Kant. Reason, duty and nation were its three pillars – Cartesian reason as the source of truth, Kantian duty understood as a categorical imperative emanating from a universal conscience, and the love of nation as taught by the republicans after the defeat of 1870, which particularly affected the daughters of Alsace. There was nothing narrow about her idealism. She showed endless curiosity towards people and works of art, so eager was she to know the true and the beautiful that lay beyond

37 Streicher taught at the *École Normale Supérieure de Sèvres*, publishing a critical edition of the seventeenth-century grammarian, Vaugelas', *Remarques sur la langue française* (Paris: Droz, 1936) ; an edition of Théophile de Viau, *Œuvres poétiques* (Geneva: Droz, 1951–58); and an edition of Pierre Corneille, *Sertorius: tragédie* (Geneva: Droz, 1959).

38 JPR: 'Jeanne Streicher – extrait de mes souvenirs', MS, PRFP.

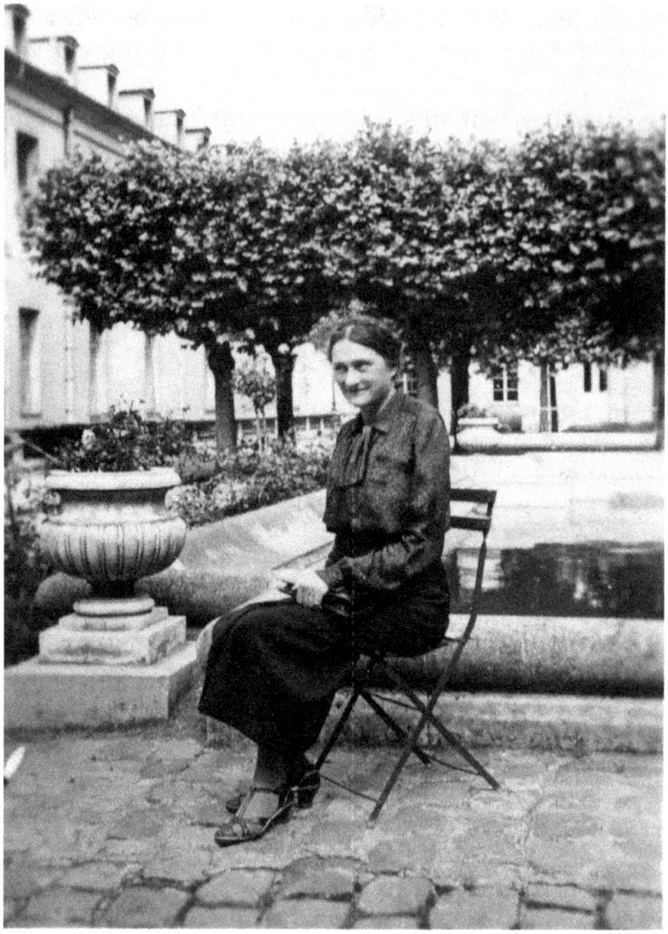

Fig 10. Jeanne Streicher at Maison Blanche c. *1930*

appearances. In her there was a mixture of puritanism and generosity that I have never found in anyone else.]

A further paradox of maintaining the secret of Jeanne's origins lay in Pascal's own character. She believed in ethical action, seeing her psychiatric work as part of a humanist project. She despised hypocrisy in others and in herself. When it became clear that Mengin would never recognize his daughter, she accepted the implicit need for secrecy with regard to Jeanne's birth, in order to protect both parents' reputations, but living this continual lie remained a source of internal conflict and shame. Nevertheless, in 1934, hearing from her brother Trajan that he was gravely ill, she wrote to him after their long period of estrangement to confess that Jeanne was indeed her biological child and General Mengin the father. Trajan responded cordially, although at the same time his reply makes clear that the tensions between him and Constance had by no means disappeared:

> De ta correspondance je vois que tu n'as pas encore rien oublié. Tu me rappelles encore des tristes moments que j'avais passés à Paris à cause des questions qui ne méritaient pas tant de chagrin et tant de bile. J'ai essayé de te faire comprendre la réalité et je n'ai pas réussi, ni même le temps n'a pu [*sic*] résoudre ce problème. C'est triste mais ce n'est pas ma faute.
>
> Quant à la petite Jeanne, je te charge de lui dire, que je l'aime et que je l'estime beaucoup. Qu'elle pense toujours à nous, quand elle se croira – Dieu la garde – seule. Tu me dis qu'elle soit [*sic*] pensive et des fois triste. Je crois qu'elle souffre moralement d'une situation que tu as mis du temps à éclaircir. [...] Tu peux lui dire que je suis son vrai oncle, et que je suis prêt à faire pour elle tout ce que je fera [*sic*] pour mon fils. Dans son enfance, Jeanne était expansive, gaie, sincère, loyale – une vraie charmante jeune fille. Il ne faut pas la faire perdre ces beaux traits de caractère.[39] C'est dangereux. Crois-moi (Corr TP & CP PRFP, 7 July 1934)

> [From your letter I see that you have still forgotten nothing. You remind me once again of the unhappy time I had in Paris because of problems that did not deserve so much grief and rancour. I have tried and failed to make you understand the truth and time has not solved this problem. It is a pity but it is not my fault.
>
> As for little Jeanne, tell her from me that I love and admire her very much. If ever she believes herself alone in the world – heaven forbid – she should remember us. You say she thinks a lot and is sometimes sad. No doubt she must suffer morally from a situation that you took so long to clarify. [...] You may tell her that I am her true uncle, and I am ready to do everything for her that I would do for my own son. When she was a child, Jeanne was outgoing, bright, sincere and loyal – a truly charming girl. You must not make her lose those fine qualities. It is a danger. Believe me.]

If Pascal did not relish being given lessons in managing a teenage daughter, she must have been relieved that Trajan – though, like her, still harbouring ancient resentments – was kindly disposed towards his niece and not shocked by her revelation. To say that he would do everything for her that he would do for his own son was probably an exaggeration. In later years, beyond welcoming Jeanne's visit to Romania, he did not offer any financial support. But from

39 Trajan's errors in French have been retained.

a patriarchal figure like Trajan these declarations of goodwill were remarkable. However, for reasons not made clear by either Pascal or her brother, the correspondence ceased at this juncture, only to be resumed by Jeanne after her mother's death.

Aside from fragments in letters, the fullest expression of Pascal's dilemmas with regard to her daughter emerges in a film script, *La Goutte de sang* [The drop of blood], written probably in 1935–36, but never produced.[40] Jean Painlevé, Director of the *Institut de Cinématographie Scientifique,* expressed interest in a screenplay that Pascal had hoped to have produced for the *Exposition Universelle,* a project Painlevé thought was not feasible in the available time. As a tribute to the realism of her scenario, however – it concerned the successful search for a reliable paternity blood test – he worried that the public might be alarmed: 'Il serait à craindre que le public ne prenne votre anticipation pour une réalité' (Corr Painlevé & CP, PRFP 15 April 1937) [There is a risk that the public might think your science fiction is a reality]. Nevertheless, Painlevé agreed to do some filming of Pascal and her patients at Maison Blanche: 'J'espère beaucoup pouvoir filmer chez vous des moments et des sujets qui vous intéresseraient' (Corr Painlevé & CP, PRFP 26 April 1937) [I hope very much to come and film at your hospital. The choice of incidents and subjects is up to you]. Evidently Pascal's worsening health made this plan impossible.

Pascal called her film-script a comedy, almost certainly an ironic subtitle, given the protagonist's death at the end. An epigraph from Renan on the title page affirms its central theme, the scientific ideal of devotion to truth, understood as a lay religion: 'Le sage n'a pas besoin de prier à ses heures, car toute sa vie est une prière' [The wise man has no need to pray at a set time, for his whole life is a prayer]. *La Goutte de sang* concerns a research biologist, François Meyran, director of the prestigious Claude Bernard scientific institute, who for the past twenty-five years has been looking for an infallible blood test to establish paternity. Meyran's zeal for this project arises from his guilt over a young woman and fellow researcher whom he seduced in his youth, then abandoned when she became pregnant. His cowardice – a word applied freely in the script to men who deny their paternity – which was based in obedience to his snobbish parents, has haunted him ever since. The first two acts explore the attitudes of scientists: on the one hand the dedicated researchers for whom science is a religion and, on the other, those who exploit their work for commercial gain, one of whom is a notorious womanizer.

40 Constance Pascal, 'La Goutte de sang', MS (PRFP 1935–36).

The play's problematic comedy of errors revolves around the ethical imperatives and consequences implicit in the scientific search for truth.

In the ranks of dedicated scientists in *La Goutte de sang* is a brilliant young researcher, Mlle Christiane Viot, respected and admired for her intellect and professional dedication, a character Pascal may have based on memories of her own youthful self. It is she who finds a trustworthy blood test to trace paternity, a discovery that Meyran believes will revolutionize social mores and eradicate hypocrisy. Errant fathers, he proclaims, will be punished: 'Les travaux biologiques sur la recherche de la Paternité et de la Filiation pourraient transformer le monde civilisé pourri de mensonges et d'erreurs' (*Goutte*, Act I, 2) [Biological research to establish paternity and filial descent could transform the civilized world, which is rotten with lies and errors]. The laboratory cynic replies, however, conveying some of Pascal's own scepticism: 'Il [Meyran] ne sait pas ce que c'est que la lâcheté des hommes et que depuis que le monde est monde, c'est le mâle qui gouverne tout' (*Goutte*, Act I, 3) [He [Meyran] does not understand the cowardice of men and the fact that since the world began it has been the male who rules everything].

With the discovery of the paternity blood test, Meyran founds the Viot Institute dedicated to reuniting children abandoned by their fathers. Under the 'Code Meyran', fathers are required to present themselves for testing in order to find their previously unacknowledged offspring. His delight with the immense success of Viot's paternity test and its social effects, however, receives a check when the latter attacks the whole enterprise for having put unacceptable constraints on human libido. Viot accuses Meyran of having destroyed human freedom:

> Pauvre Éros mutilé! Vous lui avez coupé les ailes et vous l'avez enchaîné aux nombreux articles de la nouvelle législation, basée sur l'acte de la fécondation. En rabaissant l'Amour à cet acte instinctif, vous l'avez dépouillé de son art, de sa beauté, de sa richesse sentimentale et de ses forces spirituelles. L'homme est devenu le 'bon animal' qui remplit ses devoirs et qui craint surtout vos sanctions. Vous l'obligez à supporter toute sa vie, une erreur de jeunesse, il souffre plus que l'ancien 'méchant animal' qui avait au moins la liberté, le pouvoir de faire son choix, de changer après s'être trompé, parfois de réparer. Vous avez rendu l'amour haïssable, et vous avez fait de la vertu, une mécanique affreuse! L'homme nouveau que vous avez confectionné est ridicule, anormal, malheureux. Il est perpétuellement traqué. Le mariage n'est plus qu'un bagne où les parents sont obligés d'obéir aux lois du sang du Code Meyran, même lorsqu'ils se détestent; ils vivent

comme des forçats enchaînés autour de leurs enfants malheureux. Ah ! la science, voyez-vous, ne peut pas créer une morale; elle manque de pitié, elle n'a qu'un but : la vérité froide et la justice glaciale (*Goutte*, Act III, 17).

[Poor mutilated Eros! You have clipped his wings and fettered him with this new legislation, based on the act of impregnation. In reducing Love to an instinctive act, you have stripped it of its art, its beauty, its emotional richness and its spiritual powers. Man is reduced to a 'good animal' that fulfils its duties and fears punishment above all. You force him to carry the errors of his youth with him for the rest of his life; in this he suffers more than the earlier 'bad animal', who at least had its freedom, the power to make choices, to learn from errors, sometimes to put them right. You have made love hateful and virtue into something horrible and mechanical. The new man you have concocted is ridiculous, twisted and unhappy. He is forever hounded. Marriage has been turned into a prison-house where parents are forced to obey the laws of the Code Meyran, even if they hate each other; they live chained like convicts to each other and their miserable children. Science, you must realize, cannot create a moral system; it has no pity, it has only one aim: cold truth and icy justice.]

Accused of causing more harm than good, Meyran ripostes in defence of science a force, he argues, of gradual social reform. The total freedom invoked by Viot is impossible and undesirable:

Je sais que je n'ai pas fait bondir toutes les consciences vers le sommet de l'Idéal moral; le devoir sans sanction extérieure reste toujours l'état exceptionnel. Quant à regretter la liberté en amour, c'est avouer une ignorance totale du cœur des hommes. Chère enfant, apprenez que personne n'est digne de vivre sans contrainte; personne n'est assez moral pour mériter la liberté (*Goutte*, Act III, 20).

[I know that I have not caused a great leap of the human mind towards the highest moral ideal: a sense of duty without the need for external sanctions will always be the exception. But those who deplore the loss of freedom in love demonstrate a total ignorance of the human heart. My dear child, you must realize that no one is virtuous enough to live without constraints; no one is moral enough to deserve total freedom.]

Following this exchange, Meyran discovers, in a melodramatic denouement, that Christiane Viot is his long-lost daughter. Immediately following the recognition scene he dies from the emotional shock.

Pascal's screenplay is in the French tradition of a *drame à thèse* [drama with a message]. She skilfully handles the conflicting ethical and emotional problems raised, concluding that there are no simple answers to life's dilemmas and, much as she might have wished to punish the cowardly fathers of unacknowledged children, as a writer she does not opt for utopian solutions. Her scenario reflects complex ethical issues in which the quasi-religious search for scientific truth, no matter how high-minded and dedicated, proves insufficient. 'La Science [...] ne peut pas créer une morale; elle manque de pitié' (*Goutte*, Act III, 20) [Science cannot create a moral system; it has no pity]. The majority of humankind requires moral training by habit and the constraint of law. A Kantian ethical imperative serves an elite morality, but even superior souls must renounce libidinal freedoms: 'Personne n'est assez moral pour mériter la liberté' *Goutte*, Act III, 20) [no one is moral enough to deserve total freedom].

During her tenure at Maison Blanche, Pascal had published at least eight articles and one monograph and made extensive preparations for a second on *dementia praecox*.[41] Four of these present individual case histories and four concern wider studies on dementia, schizophrenia and other psychoses. 'Chagrins d'amour et psychoses' [Sorrows of love and psychosis] is a short version of her last monograph with the same title. Three of the case histories recount experimentation with chemical shock therapies. One, 'La Joie qui guérit' [Cured by joy], records a patient's spontaneous cure and illustrates Pascal's interest in the role of the emotions in mental illness and health. One of the central themes to emerge in these works is Pascal's effort to distinguish her concept of *dementia praecox* from Bleuler's definition of schizophrenia. Her last unpublished monograph would have

41 Pascal's articles for this period in order of publication are: C. Pascal, 'Les grands syndromes psychiatriques; les démences', *Nouveau Traité de la médecine* (February, 1927), 7–125; C. Pascal, R. Abramovitz and Briau, 'Amélioration rapide d'une paralytique générale cachéctique et gâteuse par le Stovarsol associé au Demelcos (vaccin antichancrelleux de Nicolie)', *Annales médico-psychologiques,* 12e série, 1 (1928), 222–26; C. Pascal, J. Vié and P. Agasse, 'Guérison rapide d'une influencée catatonique (démence paranoïde à la suite de vaccination antityphique', *L'Encéphale,* 23e année, 10 (December 1928), 937–40; C. Pascal, J. Vié and P. Agasse, 'Impulsions homicides chez une mélancolique intermittente atteinte d'encéphalite', *L'Encéphale,* 24e année (1929), 316–22; C. Pascal and A. Deschamps, 'Psychoses de sensibilisation, allergie mentale', *Annales médico-psychologiques,* 1 (May 1931), 449–60 and 2 (June 1931), 8–20; C. Pascal, 'Chagrins d'amour et psychoses', *Le Progrès médicale,* 36 (3 September, 1932), 1513–24; C. Pascal, 'Le brouillard étiologique de la démence précoce s'est-il dissipé?', *Le Progrès médicale,* 32 (12 August, 1933); C. Pascal an J. Royer, 'La joie qui guérit', *L'Hygiène mentale,* 30, 8 (1935), 157–65.

dealt extensively with the historical background to these concepts, with differences between French and German schools of psychiatry and with the biological bases, still to be discovered, of severe mental illness.[42]

The first of these articles, 'Les démences' [Dementias] formed part of a series by various authors on 'Les Grands syndromes psychiatriques' [Major psychiatric syndromes]. Unusually in a psychiatric journal, it begins with a description of demented patients seen from the perspective of an outsider visiting a psychiatric hospital. Pascal goes beyond the cataloguing of symptoms, showing the mental patients in the abject state created by their condition, as they would appear to non-professionals:

> Lorsqu'on visite un asile d'aliénés pour la première fois, ce qui frappe avec le plus d'intensité, c'est la fréquence d'une catégorie de malades qui ont le même aspect clinique et la même activité. Agités ou déprimés, assis à la même place, accroupis dans un lit, étendus par terre, ils semblent avoir perdu tout contact affectif avec le milieu extérieur. Le regard incertain, la physionomie sans expression, atone, dénuée de surprise, de curiosité, d'aversion ou de sympathie, étrangers aux sollicitations extérieures, ces malades paraissent vivre en dehors des faits et des choses et en dehors d'eux-mêmes. Malpropres, débraillés, voraces, mangeant d'une façon répugnante, ils végètent isolés et sont réduits à une activité restreinte ('Démences', 97–8).

> [When one visits an insane asylum for the first time, what strikes one with the greatest force is the high incidence of a category of patients who all look the same clinically and are engaged in the same activity. Disturbed or depressed, whether sitting in one place, crouched on a bed or lying on the ground, they seem to have lost all emotional contact with the world around them. With wandering gaze, their expression lifeless, apathetic, lacking surprise, curiosity, aversion or sympathy, deaf to the appeals of other people, these patients seem to live outside the world of facts and things and even outside themselves. Dirty, slovenly, greedy, eating in a repulsive fashion, they vegetate, isolated and reduced to minimal activity.]

Reviewing earlier theories of dementia, Pascal particularly notes as the most significant the deterioration of the patient's affective contact.[43] The demented patient is a stranger to his or her world. Loss of feeling for others becomes part of the process leading to the disintegration of the personality. This article is the first in which she refers to Eugen Bleuler's recategorization of *dementia praecox* as

42 Constance Pascal, 'Table des Matières', for MS on '*La Démence précoce*', PRFP.

43 *Démences*, 105.

schizophrenia or psychic disassociation.[44] Noting that schizophrenia includes not only *dementia praecox*, but the most disparate psychoses, she proposes to rename it 'schizo-démence' [schizo-dementia].

The causes of early dementia attacks, which usually begin between the ages of twelve and fifteen or twenty and thirty, can only be ascertained, she suggests, through psychological means; in Freudian terms, they are probably the result of emotional conflict and repression. Pascal notes that Freud gives sexual feelings, repressed into the unconscious, a pathogenic power of the first order. Finally as regards treatment, she dissents from the view that dementia is always incurable, arguing that further work on chemical shock therapy could prove beneficial: 'La démence précoce dont l'évolution lente présente fréquemment des rémissions spontanées de longue durée, paraît susceptible de modifier sa marche fatale' ('Démences', 125) [*Dementia praecox* which, in its slow evolution, often presents long-lasting spontaneous remissions, seems capable of modifying its apparently fatal progress]. 'Les Démences' demonstrates Pascal's authority in her subject specialism and underlines her commitment to continuing research and therapeutic interventions on her patients, where appropriate, through the medium of Freud's talking cure.

The three case histories in this group of articles follow the effects of physical interventions, the so-called 'heroic therapies' used on mental illness, giving one patient a fixation abscess, another an anti-chancre drug (for syphilitic lesions), and the third, who had paranoid dementia, an anti-typhoid vaccination. In all these case histories, conclusions about cure or remission remained debatable. More interesting than these experimental and seemingly random therapies were the life histories of the patients participating in the experiments. For example, a forty-eight-year-old woman, who had lost her father to tuberculosis and whose mother and sister were both interned in a mental hospital with post-natal depression, had had four children, one of whom died at seven months. The following year she fell ill after a difficult labour and also lost her husband. Her first period of depression lasted a year followed by a twenty-year period of stability. In 1926 she again experienced a crisis of depression, made suicide attempts and became violent, attempting to strangle her daughter. The clinical interest of the case lay, for Pascal, in the atypical violence of this depressive who was also suffering from encephalitis (inflammation of the brain). The patient's great improvement over

44 Bleuler gave a paper in 1908 in which he first coined the term schizophrenia and published his *Dementia praecox, oder Gruppe der Schizophrenien* [Dementia praecox or schizophrenic groupings] in 1911.

several months led to the question of her release, problematic in view of her violent history.

In a second case, a woman patient who heard voices believed she was a medium and could hear other people's thoughts. She further believed that she was being poisoned, and was diagnosed as a case of paranoid dementia. She appeared to recover when a typhoid epidemic broke out in her ward and all patients were given anti-typhoid vaccine. When the fever induced by the vaccine abated, the patient almost completely regained her mental equilibrium. Although the immediate explanation of this cure appeared to be the anti-typhoid injection, Pascal was nevertheless cautious in her conclusion, noting that in Germany the same method had been used with variable results, not all of them benign. At Maison Blanche, where Pascal tried anti-typhoid injections on a number of patients, no similarly dramatic results occurred. Should one conclude that cure, or even amelioration, was a spontaneous event unconnected to medical intervention?

It is in light of these case histories that the article, 'La Joie qui guérit' (1935), which chronicles an unexpected remission from depression and persecution mania, reflects Pascal's constant self-questioning about her results and the effectiveness of therapy. In 'La Joie', a woman who felt she had lost her function in life now that her children were grown up was restored to sanity when her new daughter-in-law, to her delighted surprise, addressed her affectionately as 'Mother'. A woman, who had lost all sense of who and what she was, seemed to recover spontaneously when the maternal role that she felt she no longer had was restored to her:

> Notre malade jette un défi aux classifications actuelles au [*sic*] pronostic fatal. Elle nous oblige à avouer notre ignorance et à renoncer à l'évaluation des signes qui constituent l'irréversibilité. Elle nous reproche d'avoir méconnu le contenu de son délire, sa douleur morale, ses craintes inhibitrices et la vitalité de son complexe maternel. Pendant cinq ans, elle a utilisé sous nos yeux, tous les mécanismes grossiers de la psychiatrie: cris, mutisme, sitiophobie, gâtisme, incohérence du langage et des gestes, etc.; elle a organisé un délire de persécution, délire qui marque la crainte d'un danger supposé, la panique intérieure: peur immense de perdre son fils aimé. Car chez elle, le complexe maternel a été la stase affective qui a immobilisé toute son énergie, et c'est grâce à cette réserve vitale qu'elle a pu faire un saut magnifique du morbide dans le normal. Débloquée par la joie qui décharge, ses forces psychiques libérées ont abouti à la réintégration ('Joie', 162–63).

> [This patient challenges current classifications of an inevitable prognosis. She forces us to admit our ignorance and give up assessing certain symptoms as proving an irreversible decline. She shows us that we had misunderstood the content of her mania, her mental suffering, her inhibiting fears and the power of her maternal complex. For five years, under our observation, she demonstrated all the crude mechanisms of psychiatry: shouting, mutism, aversion to food, senility, incoherence of speech and gestures, etc. She displayed a coherent persecution complex, with terror of imagined dangers and inner panic: in particular, a great fear of losing her beloved son. For her maternal complex was an emotional core that was blocking all her energies, and it is thanks to that vital reserve that she was able to make the magnificent leap from illness to normality. Released by a discharge of joy, her freed psychic strength brought her to a state of reintegration.]

This case history, with its seemingly spontaneous outcome, reveals suggestive aspects about Pascal both as a clinician and as a woman. Her distrust of labelling patients, which, as we have seen, she was obliged to do in her annual reports, contrasts with her growing interest in their subjective lives. Further, this case of maternal love gone awry must have sounded alarms but also a sense of kinship with her own experience, the overwhelming desire for a child and the dangers of obsessive maternity.

Pascal's clinical research culminated in her last monograph, *Chagrins d'amour et psychoses* (1935), which represents the summation of her life experience as a psychiatrist. Calling up a host of literary, philosophical, psychiatric and psychoanalytic thinkers (for example: Bergson, Dante, Freud, Jung, Mauriac, Nietzsche, Plato, Proust, Schopenhauer and many more), her text is above all a detailed engagement with, and partial contestation of, Freudian psychoanalysis.[45] It conveys her admiration for Freud, whom she saw as revolutionizing the study of the mind, combined with a host of reservations. As she writes in her conclusion: 'Mais l'œuvre de Freud n'est pas dans ces details pédagogiques; elle est dans sa grandeur poétique et sa fécondité, car son domaine et sa valeur dépassent ceux d'une découverte scientifique' (*CAP*, 167) [The essence of Freud's

45 *Chagrins d'amour et psychoses*, though rich in cultural references, is devoid of footnotes. It is therefore not possible to be sure what texts of Freud's Pascal had read and to what extent her critique, both positive and negative, is based on secondary sources. By 1930, Freud had published all but three of his major works, so Pascal would have had access to them in German if not in French. She appears to have read *Civilization and its Discontents* [*Das Unbehagen in der Kultur*, 1930] as well as earlier works, but there are no direct quotations or referencing.

work lies not in its pedagogic details but in its poetic grandeur and richness, for its extent and value exceed those of a scientific discovery]. Her efforts to apply Freudian structures to patients on the psychotic or autistic spectrum, entirely different from Freud's own clinical practice with articulate neurotics, may account for some of her frustrations with Freud's method. On a personal level, *Chagrins* furnishes possible insights into Pascal's own passions and their sublimation.

In her appreciation of Freud, who had, she believed, opened new perspectives on mental illness and human motivation, her criticisms centred on two points, though it appears that in her discussions she tended to conflate previous theories of degeneracy and Freud's views on childhood trauma. Firstly, she argued that the past, in the form either of heredity or infantile experience, was, though important, only one factor in mental derangement. Events in adult life can equally unhinge us. People fall ill not merely by virtue of their defective constitutions (the degenerative model of much psychiatric theory) but from catastrophic events like the Great War, a point with which Freud might not have disagreed. Its shell-shocked victims who had shown no previous tendency to mental illness were a proof, she believed, that mental illness did not strike only the constitutionally weak. Secondly, she felt that Freud's description of neurosis – or, at the further end of the mental spectrum, the condition that most concerned her, psychosis – as an escape from libidinal pressures, or as a form of enjoyment of forbidden pleasures, did not take sufficient account of the genuine suffering of her patients:

> En se basant sur la suprématie de la libido, volonté de jouissance, Freud considère les névroses et les psychoses comme des paradis artificiels, vrais *lieux de plaisir* où l'amour cherche à apaiser sa faim d'amour [*sic*]. La transmutation des valeurs érotiques a créé la notion de camouflage. La libido se déplace et se déguise, revêt souvent les costumes de la préhistoire ou ceux d'un bébé (CAP, 15).
>
> [In basing his theories on the supremacy of the libido, the pleasure-seeking drive, Freud considers both the neuroses and the psychoses to be artificial paradises [*here Pascal is referring to Baudelaire's study of the effects of drugs*], true 'pleasure-houses' where love seeks to slake its hunger for love [*sic*]. The transmutation of erotic values leads to the notion of camouflage: libido, displaced and disguised, often appears dressed up in prehistoric costume or in that of a baby.]

Pascal's reservations about Freud reflect both current attitudes in French psychiatry and more practically, the difficulty of applying his theories to her psychotic patients:

> *La Folie est-elle une délivrance? La Folie est-elle une nouvelle pénitence?* Freud a ouvert la discussion. Son dogme basé sur des hypothèses, des interprétations et des analogies superficielles ne contente pas tout le monde. [...] La clinique psychiatrique réclame des preuves et des faits précis. La psychanalyse est inutilisable dans les asiles d'aliénés. Ses coups de sonde sont stériles; ils se heurtent à la muraille de l'autisme et du négativisme et reculent devant les barrages de la réticence. Freud lui-même reconnaît que la plupart des aliénés sont 'narcissiques' et incapable de transfert affectif (CAP, 16–17).

> [*Is madness a liberation? Is madness another punishment?* Freud has opened up this debate. But his dogma, based as it is on hypotheses, interpretations and superficial analogies, does not satisfy everyone. [...] Clinical psychiatry demands proofs and clear facts. One cannot practise psychoanalysis in an insane asylum. Its excavations get nowhere, they hit the blocks of autism and negativism and retreat before the barricades of resistance. Freud himself recognized that most mad people are 'narcissistic' and incapable of emotional transference.]

Pascal retained her biological model in this work, arguing for the reality of physical symptoms resulting from mental anguish. Her engagement with Freud, whom she admired for revolutionizing the map of the mind, reflects her interest not only in psychology but in wider culture. She was particularly fascinated by Freud's recourse to Greco-Roman myths, characterizing him as more of a poet than a scientist.

Chagrins d'amour opens with a reference to Morel's concept of 'folie par amour' [madness through love], the book's touchstone. Bénédict Augustin Morel (1809–1873) is remembered for his theory of degeneration and for formulating the concept of *dementia praecox* in 1860 (to be replaced in 1911 by Bleuler's new designation, schizophrenia). In *Chagrins* Pascal shows herself resistant to the determinism of Morel's degeneracy model, but invokes him for his descriptions of *folie par amour*. Eschewing the usual listing of other authorities in the history of mental medicine and the virtually obligatory scientific literature review of standard psychiatric texts, Pascal argues that novelists, poets and philosophers have understood much more about the anguish of thwarted love than have psychiatrists, who have tended to see *folie par amour* as part of some other mental malfunction. Her opening paragraph calls up the *Inferno* as a true vision of mental suffering:

> Lorsque Virgile accompagna Dante dans sa descente aux enfers, il attira son attention sur les désespérés qui crient et appellent l'amour

> perdu. On ne peut s'empêcher de penser à ces damnés d'Éros lorsqu'on écoute les plaintes des aliénés accablés par la douleur d'un amour meurtri (*CAP*, ii).
>
> [When Virgil led Dante down to Hell, he drew his attention to the despairing souls who were crying out and calling for their lost love. One cannot help but think of those souls damned by Eros when one hears the lamentations of the mad, overwhelmed by the agony of wounded love.]

Pascal argues that whereas psychiatry has shown little interest in these victims of love, psychoanalysis sees them everywhere – they are the 'refoulés' (*CAP*, 12) [repressed], who dream constantly of love. Her project in *Chagrins* is to examine the pathology of repressed sexual psychoses with their basis in the misery of unsatisfied or rejected love, raising the central question arising from her understanding of Freud's methodology and quoted above – is madness deliverance or is it a new form of punishment? For Pascal the imaginary worlds of the mad, their castles in Spain, are built on suffering. As a clinician, she emphasizes the lived experience of her patients: 'Les blessés de l'amour ne bâtissent pas toujours des châteaux sur les coteaux de la folie; ils souffrent. Chaque observation clinique est un roman d'amour déçu, une vie brisée, un chagrin qui cherche l'apaisement et qui se débat avec le souvenir' (*CAP*, 19) [These victims of love do not always build fantasy castles on the slopes of madness; they suffer. Every clinical observation reveals a tale of disappointed love, a broken life, a grief seeking peace but wrestling with memories].

Pascal's analysis of Freud centres on his pleasure principle as the supreme force of life, the cause and possibly the cure of all mental illness. Freud has demonstrated that sexual energy is not exhausted when love ends. The sorrows of love point to unused sexual capacity. She credits his theory as the first methodological attempt to link love and mental illness.[46] Freud's major achievement, she suggests, is in understanding the displacements of the libido, its metamorphoses and its symbolism. Her disquiet is with the implications of what she calls his pansexualism: 'La libido triomphante est le souffle de la vie de la psychanalyse. Freud a beau se défendre d'être pansexualiste, il a identifié la libido avec la causalité humaine' (*CAP*, 45) [The victorious libido is the lifeblood of psychoanalysis. Freud may deny he is a pansexualist, but he has identified the libido with basic human motivation]. Pascal argues that this emphasis on libidinal energy has many critics, including Jung, Adler and Steckel, who 'reprochent à

46 *CAP*, 45.

leur maître son dogmatisme orthodoxe et sa mystique inaccessible de la libido' [criticize their master for his rigid orthodoxy and the incomprehensible mysticism of his theory of the libido]. Furthermore, according to Pascal, Freudian dynamism betrays a conservative tension in which everything has already taken place in the remote past. Freud's libidinal individuals behave like Platonic archetypes, unaware of the present and the future.[47] Yet, as we have noted in her previous case histories, like Freud, she recognizes the potentially destructive force of buried memories.

In a chapter on 'mémoire affective' [affective memory], Pascal cites Ribot and Paulhan, psychologists who had shown how feelings once experienced could be revived in their entirety. But it is Proust, who best expresses her sense of memory's power:[48]

> Le 'Temps perdu' est la mort apparente des souvenirs; c'est le faux oubli, l'amnésie de Freud. Le passé est une galerie de tableaux conservés dans les ténèbres du psychisme et qui ne se modifie jamais. La création n'existe pas; tout est découvert. Le souvenir affectif domine la mort, permet de vivre hors du temps et dans l'éternité. Revenant mystérieux qui surgit du faux oubli, il fait revivre toute la tranche de vie où il a été inséré. Le temps perdu est retrouvé; il devient l'Éden du présent. [...] Proust insiste sur la résurrection parfaite du souvenir qui n'est pas un écho vague de passé mais le passé réel, vivant, ayant gardé son dynamisme ancien, la même puissance de faire frémir le corps et l'âme, enfin, un déjà senti intégral et actualisé (*CAP*, 99).

> Time is 'lost' when memories seem to be dead; it is a false oblivion, a Freudian amnesia. The past is a gallery of pictures preserved in the darkness of the psyche which never changes. There is no such thing as creation: everything is foreknown. An affective recollection overcomes death and allows one to live beyond time, eternally. It is like a mysterious ghost springing up out of that false oblivion; it brings with it the whole section of one's life in which it took place. Lost time is found again; it becomes the Eden of the present. [...] Proust insists that the recollection is perfectly restored; it is not a vague echo of the past but the living past itself, with its old dynamism unchanged and the same power to set body and soul atremble – a past sensation fully active and complete in the present.

For her patients the wounds inflicted by disastrous love are both mental and physical. Like Proust, Henri Bergson, another key figure

47 *CAP*, 50.

48 See also Danielle Bohler, *La mémoire des sensations: Proust en discussion avec une génération de philosophes* (Bordeaux, Presses Universitaires de Bordeaux, 2006).

in *Chagrins*, emphasized the creative power of the emotions. However, in morbid mental states, this very power destroys the mind:

> Le blessé d'amour est un hypermnésique affectif; sa mémoire des émotions pénibles est développée. 'Il souffre parce qu'il se souvient' (Beethoven). Le temps douloureusement vécu est continuellement retrouvé. À la charge douloureuse du passé s'ajoute la charge douloureuse du présent. Proust retrouvait l'Éden perdu alors que le blessé d'amour ressasse le désespoir, et se laisse obséder par le dégoût ou par la haine (*CAP*, 159).
>
> [The person wounded by love possesses an affective hyper-memory; his recollection of painful emotions is fully developed. 'He suffers because he remembers' (Beethoven). Past time painfully experienced is continually rediscovered. The painful burden of the present is added to the painful burden of the past. Proust rediscovered his lost Eden, whereas the person wounded by love broods endlessly over his despair and becomes obsessed with his disgust or hatred.]

In a person wounded by love in its psychotic manifestations, the will to live finds itself under threat. The *chagrin d'amour* becomes a crisis of life itself. Madness is not an escapist paradise; it is not salvation but a new mode of suffering, not the triumph of the libido but its defeat.

The difficulty with Freud's concept of infantile sexuality, for Pascal, is that it appears to support a fatalistic view of the origin of mental illness, positing, as she puts it, a kind of biological Jansenism and adding to long extant psychiatric theories of constitutional morbidity. While these are undeniably important, she believes environmental or exogenous factors, explain much of the origin and progress of pathological states and offer hope of change.[49] While Freud's work is of immense and enduring value in having revolutionized the debate on sexuality, yet she sees him as fundamentally a pessimist for whom civilization is necessarily opposed to the pleasure principle. However, in her conclusion, Pascal differs from Freud only in emphasis, defending the right of civilization to demand sacrifices from its members whilst recognizing the libidinal price to be paid. She concludes that laws entailing the sacrifice of sexual desires are necessary for civilization to flourish and represent moral progress. Speaking from clinical and personal experience, Pascal concludes that love should not be the highest goal to which we aspire:

> L'amour trompe la soif de l'absolu et de la beauté; il ne fournit que des illusions vite perdues. [...] Dynamisme sans élévation, il est incapable

49 *CAP*, 162–3.

> de réaliser les valeurs les plus hautes. Il est nocif parce qu'il remue la vase de l'inconscient, éveille les instincts possessifs, agressifs et destructifs et mêle la douleur et la peur au bonheur éphémère (*CAP*, 66–67).
>
> [We long for beauty and the absolute; love seems to satisfy this longing, but all it gives us are illusions that are speedily lost. [...] Love is action without elevation; it is incapable of realizing the highest values. It can only harm us, for it stirs up the sludge of the unconscious, arouses possessive, aggressive and destructive instincts and adds pain and fear to short-lived happiness.]

Humanity will not be saved by sexual liberation, quite the reverse – a contention that appealed to one of the book's contemporary reviewers, who saw Pascal as a traditional moralist, striving to contain her patients' unbridled sexual passions.[50] 'La liberté sexuelle n'est-elle pas une grave erreur de la psychanalyse? La psychose guette les sous-hommes chaque fois qu'on n'a su limiter leurs appétits' (*CAP*, 165) [One of the serious errors of psychoanalysis is sexual liberation. Psychosis lies in wait for weak individuals who fail to control their appetites]. When read in conjunction with '*La Goutte de sang*', *Chagrins d'amour et psychoses* strikes a similar note of controlled pessimism: 'personne n'est assez moral pour mériter la liberté' (*Goutte*, Act III, 20) [No one is moral enough to deserve total freedom].

During the 1930s Pascal wrote a paper in response to a Dr Daumezon, who had asked her for guidance about doing research in psychiatry. Georges Daumezon (1912–79) was at the beginning of his career when he contacted Pascal. After a law degree in 1932, he gained his doctorate in medicine in 1935. As a hospital director he developed institutional psychotherapy. Becoming head of the Henri-Rousselle section of the Sainte-Anne Psychiatric Hospital, he created the Centre psychiatrique d'orientation et d'accueil. Pascal's reply to the young man sums up her own career, renders a devastating judgement on aspects of her profession, her *credo* as a psychiatrist, her views on psychiatric training and what she saw as the possibilities as well as the limitations of psychiatric practice:

> Pour réaliser une carrière de recherches après de nombreuses années d'études psychiatriques, il faut garder l'esprit jeune, curieux, naïf et avant tout de se débarrasser de l'acquis livresque, celui qui ne repose que sur des théories, assemblages de mots. [...] Que chercher? Comment? Tout d'abord, vous instruire. Il faut arriver, à

50 Georges Demay, 'Chagrins d'amour et psychoses' *L'Aliéniste français, bulletin de l'association amicale des médecins des établissements publics d'aliénés* (July 1935), 414–15.

force d'interroger les malades, au niveau du sage: savoir l'immensité de l'inconnu et les limites pauvres du connu. […] Que chercher? Le grand mystère de la pensée normale et celui de la pensée morbide. Pas d'herbier de maladies mentales. […] Mais établissez petit à petit l'herbier des malades. Étudiez les aliénés avant l'aliénation mentale. Par tous les moyens les plus simples: l'observation, la comparaison. Je déplore chez mes collègues la méconnaissance totale de l'aliéné; avant tout, on lui colle une étiquette avec un mot grec et on le poursuit ainsi toute sa vie. […] Il y a des aliénistes qui sont plus nuisibles que les cataclysmes dévastateurs. Ils détruisent tout en voulant construire. La psychanalyse a eu du bon; elle nous a livré le jeu de la vie émotionnelle. Mais à bas Œdipe! […] C'est en vieillissant qu'on arrive au stade du doute mais si l'esprit a gardé sa vitalité, on sait aussi que l'aliéné est un être passionnant; il vous livre chaque jour un monde de faits qui avivent la curiosité. Je suis restée curieuse de tout le mystère de leurs pensées, je les écoute avec plus de dévotion que lorsque j'étais jeune. […] Je n'accepte pas le Jansénisme biologique ou psychopathologique. Les constitutions et l'hérédité fixe sont des non-sens, des théories qui complètent notre ignorance. Tout est modifiable. […] Les aliénés renferment le grand mystère de la pensée, sa naissance et sa mort. […] Le fonds mental des malades est plus intéressant que le comportement à moins qu'on possède le fil d'Ariane qui va de l'acte à la cause.[51]

[To achieve a career in research after many years of psychiatric study, one must keep one's mind youthful, enquiring and naive, and above all one must get rid of all traces of book-learning, which is based on theories – mere collections of words. […] What to research on, and how? First of all, *find out for yourself.* Talking to patients, asking them questions, is the only path to wisdom: that way you will understand the immensity of what is unknown and the feeble limits of what is known. […] What to research on? The great mystery of the normal mind and the diseased mind. Don't try to create a herbarium of mental illnesses […] but, little by little, create a herbarium of the mentally ill. Study mad people before you try to study madness, and do it by the simplest means – observation and comparison. Many of my colleagues are woefully ignorant of their patients; before they do anything else, they slap on a label with a Greek word on it and it's around the patient's neck for the rest of his life […] Some psychiatrists do more harm than a devastating cataclysm. They destroy everything, thinking they are building something. Psychoanalysis has much that is valuable in it; it has shown us the play of emotional life. But forget Oedipus! [...] As one grows older one learns to doubt, but if the mind has kept its vitality one knows also that the insane are fascinating

51 Corr CP & Georges Daumezon, médecin des hôpitaux psychiatriques (PRFP *c.* 1935–36).

> people; every day they open to us a world of phenomena that inspire curiosity. I am just as curious as I ever was to understand the mystery of how they think; I listen to them with more dedication than when I was young. [...] I have no time for biological or psychopathological Jansenism. Fixed constitutions and heredity are nonsense – theories that just confirm our ignorance. Everything is changeable. [...] The insane hold the key to the great mystery of thought, its birth and its death. The inner mental world of patients is more interesting than their behaviour, unless one is in possession of the Ariadne's thread that leads from the act to the cause.]

This remarkable document, which expresses Pascal's severe reservations about the arrogance and abuse of power of some in her profession ('There are psychiatrists who are more harmful than devastating cataclysms'), the importance of clinical observation over abstract theory, her continuing fascination with mental life and her enduring optimism about the possibility of change and mental renewal, demonstrates her vitality, intellectual curiosity and professional engagement in what proved to be the last stage of her career. Her energy seemed unabated; her prominence in her profession assured. So it was that the recurrence of her cancer in 1937, which she faced with public stoicism, filled her with understandable anguish.

8. Conclusion

Throughout her adulthood, Pascal had led a peripatetic existence, first as a student and then as a psychiatrist transferring from one asylum to another. At Clermont, Prémontré, Châlons and Moisselles her conditions of employment provided her with a house in or near the hospital grounds. In spite of all the advantages of proximity to her work, as well as the financial assistance of a rent-free tied house, she had, most painfully at Clermont, felt the pressure of institutional life. In 1934, at Maison Blanche, Pascal, who by now was earning 58,000 francs a year (having started there at 28,000 francs in 1927) and who must have amassed some savings, bought an almost derelict farmhouse on the outskirts of the village of Chantemanche in the upper Marne Valley, about an hour by train from Maison Blanche.[1]

Here she and Jeanne finally had their own home during the holidays. The house, a rambling structure set in an orchard, looked out over fields. In spring, with the apple trees in bloom and the sun shining, Chantemanche would have reminded Pascal of her Romanian childhood on the small family estate at Pistesi, where Trajan still farmed. During the next three years, she spent as much time there as she could, modernising the property, installing running water and sanitation and filling it with furniture collected over the years: great walnut presses and bookshelves for her multitudes of books, oak tables and brass bedsteads. The house, its setting and furniture, remains today as in a time-warp, scarcely changed from the 1930s. It was kept by Jeanne throughout her life as a holiday home, and crucially as a site to commemorate her mother. An enormous pleasure to herself and to her daughter, Pascal's house purchase was also a prudent move; it had allowed her, at a time of

1 État des Services de Mademoiselle le Docteur Pascal, Médecin-chef de 1ère classe; Maison Blanche DACP, lists Pascal's salary increases over the course of her career. I wish to thank Michel Caire for making these documents available to me.

growing economic uncertainty, to leave Jeanne an asset in property. Chantemanche also embodied her quest for a private space.

Since the end of 1936, Pascal had kept diagnostic notes on her own condition. Near-illegible as these are, they reveal that she feared a recurrence of cancer from her new symptoms – trembling, pain and weight loss.[2] In June 1937, she began to suffer bouts of terrible pain. Until that summer she had kept up her punishing work schedule as well as supervising her daughter's studies in history. Also in 1937, fearing the spread of fascism, she joined the Socialist Party.[3] Only five months before her illness worsened, in a letter to an unnamed Spanish colleague dated 29 January, she still seemed in good spirits, sending him an article he had requested about her psychiatric career and expressing her admiration for the Spanish republican cause: 'Je vous félicite de votre bel enthousiasme, j'espère que vous arriverez à réhabiliter la république espagnole; je le souhaite de tout mon cœur, je partage vos idées'[I congratulate you on your splendid enthusiasm: I hope you will succeed in rebuilding the Spanish Republic; I wish it with all my heart, I share your ideals] (CP to unknown correspondent, PRFP 29 January, 1937). In the New Year she had written to her former mentor at Ville Evrard, Paul Sérieux, now ageing and unwell, but delighted, he said in his reply, to be reminded of the happy year 1907 when she worked under him. He added: 'En vous adressant mes souhaits sincères pour 1937, laissez-moi vous conseiller de ne point vous abandonner au découragement, de supporter avec indifférence les ennuis administratifs, et de vous remettre à la rédaction de votre livre sur la démence précoce' (Corr Paul Sérieux & CP, PRFP January 1937) [In sending you my sincere good wishes for 1937, let me advise you not to give way to despondency; you should ignore administrative annoyances and go back to your work on the new edition on *dementia praecox*]. In May she was well enough to compose a long reply to Dr Édouard Toulouse who, as Technical Sanitary Adviser to the Minister of Public Health and recognizing Pascal's expertise, had asked her for advice on the organization of psychiatric 'open' clinics in the Seine region.[4] Thereafter, Pascal's illness worsened inexorably. A former intern, Jacques Archaimbault, wrote: 'Vos souffrances me désolent; il est injuste que la douleur s'acharne sur ceux qui ont fait lutte contre elle pour les autres' (Corr CP & Jacques Archaimbault, PRFP 1937) [I am so sorry to hear about your sufferings; it is unjust

2 JPR, 'Début de la maladie', 1936–37, PRFP.

3 Constance Pascal, Carte d'Adhérent, Parti Socialiste et Feuille de Cotisations, PRFP 1937.

4 JPR, 'Début de la maladie', 1936–37, PRFP.

that pain should attack those who have fought so hard against it for others]. Pascal hid the severity of her illness from her colleagues as long as possible and did not even contact her brother Trajan when she knew she was dying. Her efforts to lead a normal life during her cancer's progress are recorded in Jeanne Pascal Rees's account of her mother's last months:

> Nous visitons l'Exposition Universelle à Paris. Depuis longtemps elle admire l'œuvre des Soviets pour les enfants handicapés, abandonnés. Mais sur le cahier des visiteurs elle écrit; 'Pourquoi ces procès, ces exécutions, ces violences?' À Maison Blanche elle reçoit un Congrès International de psychiatres venus la saluer. De mi-juillet à octobre C.P. eut congé de maladie. Elle s'affaiblit. Elle va de son lit à son bureau au 1e étage, pour travailler. Les neurologues se succèdent. C.P. semble vouloir explorer les diagnostiques possibles par conscience professionnelle et pour m'éviter la tristesse de la savoir mourir. Elle se sait condamnée. Le 17 juillet, jour où j'ai 21 ans et où cessa sa tutelle, elle m'ouvre un compte bancaire et y transfert tout ce qu'elle peut. Elle reçoit peu mais accueille Edmund Rees, venu pour l'Exposition. Au mois d'octobre la doctoresse Chassigneux m'écrit qu'il n'y a plus de doute: C.P souffre d'une métastase du cancer de 1928. Sans mentionner le cancer, C.P. m'autorise à prévenir J.S. [Jeanne Streicher]. Celle-ci la rassura, bien que je suis majeure, qu'elle s'occupera de moi.[5]
>
> [We visited the *Exposition Universelle* in Paris. She had long admired the Soviet Union for its work with handicapped and abandoned children. But at the Soviet pavilion, she wrote in the visitors' book: 'Why these trials, these executions, this violence?' At Maison Blanche she received a delegation from the International Congress of Psychiatrists, who had come to honour her. From mid July to October she took sick leave and grew ever weaker. She would go from her bed to her study to work. One neurologist after another came to see her. C.P. seemed to want to try all possible diagnoses both out of a sense of professional responsibility and to spare me the sadness of knowing she was dying. She knew this was the end. On 17 July, the day I turned twenty-one and was no longer a minor, she opened a bank account for me and transferred everything she could into it. She received almost no one, but welcomed Edmund Rees who had come to Paris for the *Exposition Universelle*. In October, C.P.'s doctor wrote to me saying that there was no longer any doubt: C.P. was suffering from a metastasis of the cancer that was first diagnosed in 1928. Without mentioning the cancer, C.P. authorized me to inform J.S. [*Jeanne Streicher*]. The latter reassured her that although I was of age she would look after me.]

5 Jeanne Pascal Rees, 'Maladie et mort de C.P., June–December, 1937', MS, PRFP 2003.

Although she did not die until 21 December 1937, Pascal had drawn up detailed plans for her funeral four years earlier, in a letter addressed to her daughter, dated 1933. She had long dreaded the return of her cancer. The document, in a handwritten scrawl, must have been shocking for Jeanne to read:

> Mes dernières volontés.
>
> Si le malheur arrive, voici ce qu'il faudra faire.
>
> Ne pas pleurer, c'est inutile.
>
> S'occuper de mes obsèques très rapidement: un cercueil solide pour que les vers n'entrent pas dedans.
>
> Si ceci n'est pas trop cher: achetez un caveau pour nous deux dans un cimetière de campagne proche où tu peux venir me voir de temps en temps.
>
> Aucun frais d'enterrement: défense absolue de parade, de corbillard, de chevaux empanachés, de discours, de pleurs, de couronnes. Rien – Rien que ma voiture qui ira vite me déposer dans le Trou. N'invitez pas les soi-disant amis; je ne veux que Jeanne Streicher et toi.
>
> Tu dois faire tuer les chiens pour qu'ils ne souffrent pas.
>
> Toi? Je te conseille de vivre avec les étrangers. Je n'ai pas d'amis, pas de famille. Je te laisse seule. Débrouille-toi. Vive. Tu es intelligente, tu as droit à la vie comme les autres.
>
> Adieu
>
> C. Pascal (30 August 1933 PRFP).
>
> [My last wishes
>
> If the worst happens, this is what you must do.
>
> Do not weep; there is no point.
>
> Arrange my funeral as quickly as possible: a solid coffin so that the worms cannot get in.
>
> If it is not too expensive, buy a vault for us both in a country graveyard nearby where you can come and see me from time to time.
>
> Do not spend any money on the funeral. I absolutely forbid any parade or procession; no hearse, horses with plumes, speeches, tears or wreaths. Nothing, nothing but my own car to take me quickly and put me in the Ground. Do not invite my so-called friends; I want no one but Jeanne Streicher and you.
>
> You must have the dogs killed so that they do not suffer.
>
> As for you, I advise you to live among strangers. I have no friends and no family. I am leaving you alone. You will have to manage. Live. You are intelligent, you have as much right to life as anyone else.
>
> Farewell.
>
> C. Pascal]

This document encapsulates a sense of Pascal's despair at her probable untimely death, her anxieties for Jeanne and her sense of social isolation. Yet she had numerous colleagues, good friends among the staff at the hospital and eminent acquaintances in psychiatry and the political world. Letters from colleagues and hospital staff express the greatest affection. The bleakness of her envisaged funeral appears as a kind of self-mortification. She wanted no recognition of her professional role, of her ground-breaking work as a woman in psychiatry,[6] or of her great contribution to the care and education of handicapped children, and of course nothing about her private life. It was as though she was resolved on total obliteration, by denying both her life's achievements and any public knowledge of her true maternity. Jeanne Pascal Rees recalled this terrible time, quite without self-pity, though she must have been overwhelmed before a future without her mother, who had been the rock of her existence. There were to be no elegiac final scenes:

> Il faut écarter l'image de la famille et des amis au chevet de la malade. Il y a à côté de moi le petit groupe des infirmières, des malades qui s'occupent de la maison, des chiens qui errent désolés. JS venait régulièrement. Pas de prêtre. J'ai écarté brutalement le curé catholique de Neuilly: C.P. est d'origine orthodoxe et libre penseuse. En fait, elle fait seule face à la mort, sans se plaindre, soucieuse du sort d'autrui. [...] Je crois que tout le monde avait l'impression d'assister à une tragédie; celle qui vivait, une femme en pleine force, soudainement abattue par un mal incurable et des souffrances atroces. Cela laissait sans voix et comme paralysé. [...] C.P. meurt dans la matinée du 21 décembre en ma présence et celle des infirmières. J.S. arrivée trop tard, me dit de prendre toutes les décisions (JPR, 'Maladie et mort').

> [Forget all about images of family and friends gathered around the sickbed. Apart from me there was the small group of nurses and the patients who looked after the house and the dogs wandering about miserably. Jeanne Streicher came regularly. There was no priest. I sent the Catholic curé of Neuilly packing: C.P. had been brought up Orthodox but was a freethinker. In fact, she faced death alone, without complaint, thinking only of the future of others. [...] I believe everyone felt as though they were watching a tragedy: an active woman in her prime, struck down by an incurable illness, suffering horribly. We were all silenced and as if paralysed. [...] C.P. died on the morning of 21st December; I was there, as were the nurses. J.S., who arrived too late, told me to take all necessary decisions.]

6 To her Spanish correspondent Pascal played down her importance as the 'first woman in psychiatry', PRFP, 29 January 1937.

In a terse announcement, the Director of Maison Blanche, following Pascal's instructions, alerted the hospital staff as to the funeral arrangements:

> Le Directeur de l'hôpital psychiatrique de Maison Blanche fait part du décès de Mademoiselle le Dr Pascal, Médecin-chef de la 3e Section.
>
> Les agents qui désireraient s'incliner devant le cercueil pourront le faire dans la journée du 22 décembre, à l'amphithéâtre de l'établissement où le corps sera transporté. Suivant la volonté expresse de la défunte, aucun cortège ne devra suivre le convoi funéraire, de même qu'on est prié de n'apporter ni fleurs, ni couronnes.[7]
>
> [The Director of the psychiatric hospital of Maison Blanche announces the death of Dr Pascal, *Médecin Chef* of the 3rd Section. Staff wishing to pay their respects may visit the coffin during the day of 22 December in the hospital amphitheatre, where the body will be brought. Following the express wishes of the deceased, no procession will follow the funeral cortege; similarly, no flowers or wreaths, by request.]

Jeanne Rees recalls her mother's final departure from Maison Blanche:

> L'enterrement, jeudi 23 décembre. Dans la grande salle de la Morgue de l'asile, les assistants sont en demi-cercle autour du cercueil. Pas de fleurs, pas de musique, pas de discours. J.S. et moi nous sommes debout à l'entrée. Chacun vient nous serrer la main — silence. Puis dans l'auto nous suivons le corbillard dénudé trainait par un seul cheval. Au cimetière J.S. et moi, nous sommes seules et silencieuses devant la fosse où on descend le cercueil (JPR, 'Maladie et mort').
>
> [The funeral, Thursday 23 December. In the great hall of the asylum morgue, people gathered in a semi-circle around the coffin. No flowers, no music, no speeches. J.S. and I were standing by the door. One by one they came to shake our hands – in silence. Then in the car we followed the bare hearse drawn by a single horse. At the cemetery J.S. and I stood at the graveside, alone and silent, watching the coffin lowered into the ground.]

Jeanne Rees believed that her mother had suffered deeply from the perceived need to keep secret both her adulterous liaison with General Mengin and her daughter's birth. Although she had managed, by adopting her to create the fiction that her own child was a war orphan of unknown parentage, Pascal had never told Jeanne of her adoption. The latter had always believed Pascal was her natural

7 Note by the Director Maison Blanche to all staff, 21 December 1937, copy courtesy of Dr Michel Caire, Maison Blanche.

mother, only discovering the ruse of her adoption after her mother's death.[8] After the funeral, Jeanne left Maison Blanche to live with Mlle Streicher who, devoted to her friend's memory, saw it as her task to shelter Pascal's daughter and ensure that she passed the *agrégation* examination in history; the highly competitive *agrégation* was the only entry-way to a career teaching in French *lycées*. Strich, as her students called her, was a formidable figure:

> Grande, mince, un peu voûtée à force de rester penchée sur les livres, son visage buriné rappelait celui de Voltaire dont elle avait les yeux vifs et pénétrants. Deux nattes soigneusement fixées encerclaient sa tête; le menton légèrement galoche créait une sorte de ligne de démarcation avec le reste du corps où rien de saillant n'apparaissait car la poitrine semblait fort plate. J'ai revu cette même silhouette sérieuse et concentrée dans les femmes que peignait les le Nain, picards eux aussi.[9] (JPR, 'Recollections of Jeanne Streicher', MS, PRFP 2003)
>
> [Tall, thin, a little stooped, due to a life spent bending over books, her deeply lined face reminded one of Voltaire, whose sharp, penetrating eyes she also had. Her hair was carefully plaited and fixed in two bands around her head. Her somewhat prominent chin formed a kind of demarcation line from the rest of her body in which nothing else stood out, as her chest was very flat. I have seen this same serious and concentrated form in women painted by the le Nain brothers, who were also from Picardy.]

Though Jeanne had specialized in philosophy for her baccalaureate, when she transferred to the *Lycée Henri IV* to prepare the *agrégation* she switched to history, finding the philosophy taught at *Henri IV* too arid and mechanistic. By 1935 she was enrolled as a student at the *Faculté des Lettres* and in receipt of a student allowance.[10] Her two major bereavements, the deaths of her father and her mother within five years, the obligation, carried over from her mother to continue her studies, and the pressure from Mlle Streicher to succeed could have constituted a crushing burden. Nevertheless, under Strich's

8 Pascal's 'identification file (Notes Signalétiques) from Maison Blanche listing all her previous posts, includes under the heading 'situation de famille' the following information: 'Célibataire. Enfant adopté le 6 Février 1924 – Tribunal Civil de la Seine' Maison Blanche DACP.

9 Le Nain was the name of three brothers: Antoine (1588–1648), Louis (1593–1645), Mathieu (1607–77), French painters of genre, peasant and mythological scenes, born in Laon, Picardy.

10 Certificate of enrolment, Université de Paris: Faculté des Lettres, Maison Blanche DAPC 3 March 1936.

somewhat Spartan regime and firm tutorial guidance, she plunged into work, buckling down to a ferocious programme of study.

Soon after her mother's funeral, Jeanne wrote to her Romanian relations to inform them of Pascal's death, hoping as well to discover the source of their family disagreements. Her first letter was addressed to her uncle, General Trajan Pascal, whose address she found among her mother's papers. Unsure whether he knew about her origins, she made clear her own illegitimate status and General Mengin's paternity, as well as his refusal to acknowledge her legally.[11] Trajan replied on 10 March 1938 in the most cordial terms and, while he said he regretted the past, he denied any reason on his side for the estrangement between him and his sister:

> Votre lettre, par laquelle vous m'annoncez la mort de votre mère et ma sœur, nous a causé une douloureuse surprise et énormément de peine. Une femme supérieure comme elle, avec sa grande et belle intelligence, vaste culture et expérience, ne méritait pas une fin si douloureuse. Je regrette et je regretterai toute ma vie cette froideur que nous a éloignés – frère et sœur – mais en examinant ma conscience, je ne vois pas le moindre motif qui la justifiait (Corr TP & JP, Pitesti, PRFP 10 March 1938).
>
> [Your letter informing us of the death of your mother, my sister, came as a shock and caused us much pain and sorrow. She was an exceptional woman, with a great and fine intelligence, vast culture and experience, and she did not deserve such a painful end. I regret and will regret all my life the coldness that came between us as brother and sister, but in examining my conscience, I find not the slightest motive to justify it.]

He recalled his sojourn in Paris in 1920–21 when he had played with little Jeanne who, he said, young as she was, had been his French teacher, correcting his grammatical errors and pronunciation: 'Je vous ai tenu sur mes genoux et nous avons lu ensemble de petits contes, dans le petit appartement que ma sœur occupait à Charenton après la guerre' [You used to sit on my lap and together we would read little stories, in the little apartment where my sister lived at Charenton after the war].

Her cousin Ion, whom she had known as a child, was now married, had a doctorate in law from the University of Bucharest and was completing a second doctorate in political economy in Berlin. Ion's wife, Valérie, was a chemist. Trajan added, with parental pride:

11 Much of the content of Jeanne's letters to her uncle and cousin, which do not survive, can be inferred from their replies; see correspondence with the Pascal family after the death of Constance Pascal, PRFP 1938–1945.

'Comme vous voyez, une famille d'intellectuels' [As you can see, we are a family of intellectuals]. With regard to Jeanne's illegitimate status, Trajan dismissed the problem as relating to outmoded prejudices:

> Tout se résume à une question de 'forme' qui pour nous tous n'a aucune importance. Filiation, adoption etc., c'est la même chose. Vous êtes pour nous tous la fille de ma sœur. C'est tout. Quant au Général Mengin, je ne m'explique pas sa conduite. Je l'ai toujours connu *gentleman*. En lisant votre lettre, je m'explique la torture morale de ma sœur et même sa conduite envers nous. Je n'ai su que vous êtes sa fille légitime[12] que le jour où elle me l'a fait connaître – c'est-à-dire il y a quatre ans sur mon lit d'hôpital. Elle a commencé sa lettre par 'je t'ai menti' et elle l'a finie par un 'pardon'. C'était tout à fait inutile. Il n'était pas besoin de me mentir ni de me demander pardon. Je vous ai toujours aimée comme sa fille légitime (Corr TP & JP, Pitesti, PRFP 8 May 1938).
>
> [All this is just a matter of form; it does not matter to us. Filiation, adoption etc. – it's the same thing. As far as we are concerned, you are my sister's child, that's all. As for General Mengin, I cannot understand his behaviour. I had always found him a proper 'gentleman' [*English in the original*]. Reading your letter, I understand better what my sister went through and even how she behaved towards us. I only knew you were her true daughter when she told me – that was four years ago, during my illness in hospital. She began her letter by saying 'I lied to you', and ended saying 'Forgive me'. Both those things were unnecessary. There was no need to lie to me or to ask for my forgiveness. I have always loved you as her legitimate daughter.]

The family correspondence continued, and includes a series of remarkable letters between the two cousins only interrupted by the war. These convey Ion's pleasure at discovering a near relation with whom he feels in close sympathy, his veneration for his distinguished aunt, whom he remembers from his childhood, his admiration for French culture and the French language (which he wrote beautifully), personal reflections about the frustrations attendant on seeking a meaningful career in Romania and descriptions of the social world in which his family moved. Yearning for life in the West, Ion suffered from the realization that, as a Romanian, his economic future lay in Germany. At the same time he demonstrates a strong spirit of Romanian nationalism, which emerges in his correspondence as depression alternating with romantic elation. His letters to Jeanne

12 Trajan Pascal appears to mean that Jeanne was Pascal's biological daughter rather than legitimate in law.

resemble love-letters – not to her, but to an imagined world and future in which he could not share.

The first of these, dated 13 May 1938 and some sixteen pages long, laments the past where the families had been alienated, but expressed hopes for a renewed and durable friendship with his cousin:

> Votre réponse à la lettre de mon père fut pour nous tous une vraie joie. Elle efface d'un trait un passé qui nous a tous fait souffrir. Que de fois n'ai-je moi-même maudit ces malentendus dont je ne connaissais même pas la raison mais qui ont pourtant séparé pendant tant d'années des êtres qui en réalité – j'en suis sûr – étaient capables de s'aimer et de se comprendre. Moi-même, j'en ai souffert profondément et, sans presque la connaître, j'aimais ma tante, votre mère, et je l'admirais. Elle représentait pour moi un idéal, la passion du travail, la forme la plus noble de l'ambition qui ne trouve son apaisement que dans le travail désintéressé – et j'ai toujours profondément regretté d'en avoir été séparé par de stupides malentendus dont nous ne connaîtrons probablement jamais les vraies origines. C'est là un côté tragique de l'existence de nos parents, que nous n'avons pas à juger, mais qui n'en aura pas moins influence sur notre vie (Corr Ion Pascal &JP, Berlin, PRFP 13 May 1938).

> [Your reply to my father's letter was a great joy to us all. In one stroke it cancelled out the past. How many times have I cursed that misunderstanding which made all of us unhappy, whose cause was unknown to me and yet which I could see was keeping apart two people who, in reality, I'm sure, were made to love and understand each other. I suffered deeply from it myself and, even though I scarcely knew her, I loved my aunt, your mother, and admired her. For me she stood for an ideal – the passion for work, the most noble form of ambition which is only fulfilled in disinterested labour. I have always deeply regretted being kept from her by stupid misunderstandings whose true origins we will probably never know. That is a tragic aspect of our parents' lives, which it is not for us to judge, but it has had an effect on our lives as well.]

When, in 1938–39, Jeanne's letters expressed doubts about her ability to pass her *agrégation* examination, Trajan offered encouragement, praising her undoubted abilities and the debt of intellectual brilliance that she owed to her Pascal inheritance:

> Vous possédez, chère amie, une force incontestable de raison et une manière inégalable d'exposer une question, les deux résultat, sans doute, d'une éducation supérieure et d'une préparation pour la vie que rarement une jeune fille de votre âge soit en état de posséder. [...] J'ai fait cette constatation d'après vos lettres qui sont vraiment des pages de bon sens, de discernement, d'un solide jugement avec

> un pessimisme qui n'est pas toujours à sa place. […] Courage, chère Jeanne, tâchez de jeter par-dessus le bord toute idée préconçue, ayez confiance dans vos possibilités et pensez à votre maman. […] N'oubliez jamais que vous êtes la fille de votre maman qui comme jeune femme a été obligée dans un pays étranger de se forger une carrière qu'elle animait avec tant de force (Corr TP & JP, Pitesti, PRFP 23 April 1939).

> [My dear young friend, you have indisputable powers of reasoning and an unrivalled gift for presenting a question – both the result, no doubt, of an excellent education and a preparation for life to which few girls of your age have access. […] I have found the evidence for this in your letters, which truly are full of good sense, wisdom and sound judgement, combined with a pessimism that is often out of place. […] Have courage, dear Jeanne: try to cast off all preconceived ideas; have confidence in your own capacities and think of your mama. […] Never forget that you are the daughter of someone who, as a young woman, found herself in a foreign country where she had to build up the career that she later sustained with such fortitude.]

Running through this correspondence is the pride her Romanian relatives took in Constance Pascal's distinguished career, a pride of which, ironically, she seems never to have been aware. The sense of being undervalued by her own family is one of the abiding themes of her surviving letters.

Jeanne Pascal passed her examination in history in May 1939, coming fourth out of three hundred candidates. It was a brilliant result. In July Trajan sent his congratulations, adding that their family had never taken her doubts seriously.[13] That summer she took a trip to Romania to visit her uncle, aunt and cousin. Trajan's avuncular persona in his letters is somewhat belied by Jeanne's actual impression of him. In many respects he was a traditional Romanian landowner, with authoritarian attitudes, especially towards women, a trait that had antagonized his sister. Jeanne thought that his wife, Marie, of whom Constance had been very fond, was terrorized by her husband, as were the household servants and peasants working on the estate.[14]

On her return to France, now an *agrégée* and qualified teacher, Jeanne was appointed to the *lycée* of Lisieux, and subsequently to posts at Rouen and Versailles. Then in 1945, after the Liberation of France, she received a letter from her former English tutor, Edmund Rees, who was stationed in Belgium with the RAF, enquiring after her

13 Corr TP & JP, Pitesti, PRFP, 16 July 1939.

14 IJPR, 15–16 July 2002.

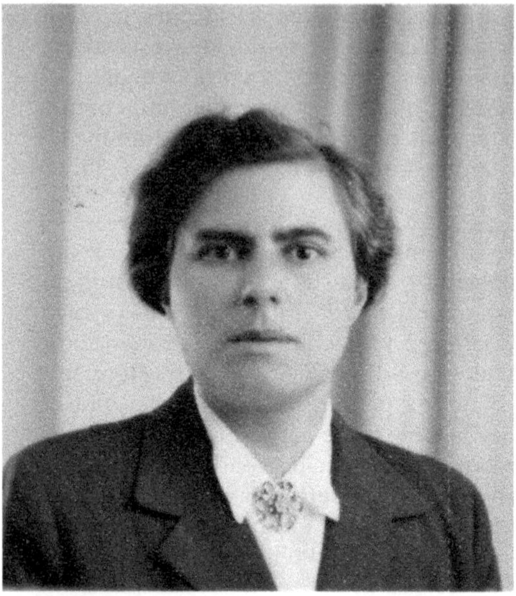

Fig 11. *Jeanne Pascal* c. 1945

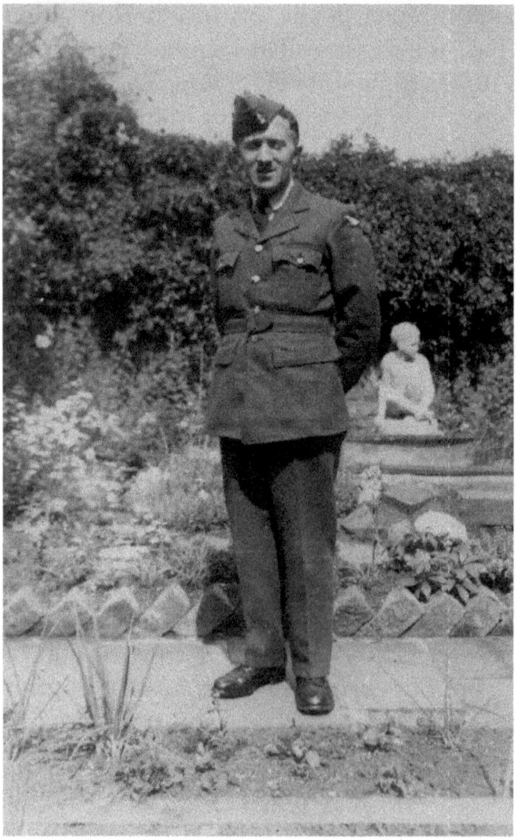

Fig 12. *Edmund Rees in British air force uniform* c. 1945

welfare and asking whether there was anything she needed. Jeanne replied that since, thanks to war shortages, she only had *sabots* as footwear, she would very much like a pair of shoes and sent him her shoe size. Edmund supplied these and later – as she told the story – she always said: 'Il m'a pris par les pieds' (IJPR, 15–16 July 2002) [He wooed me by my feet]. The friendship, begun when Edmund Rees was her teacher and she an unwilling teenage student of English, ended with their marrying in 1946 and moving permanently to England. Constance Pascal's fears for her daughter's future, fortunately, were unrealized. Jeanne Pascal Rees and her husband taught in London for many years, moving on retirement to Oxford, where their daughter was a medical consultant. Mme Rees re-established relations with her Romanian family after the war, managing several visits over the years.

The Romanian Pascals survived reasonably well under the Ceauşescu regime. At the end of the war, Ion, his wife Valérie and their young son, when liberated from the Germans (they had been interned as enemy aliens in Germany in 1944 when Romania went over to the Allies), were sent to Italy but ultimately returned to Romania to look after their ageing parents. In spite of his doctorate in economics, under the Romanian communist regime and owing to his war record of working in a Romanian diplomatic mission to Germany, Ion was demoted to factory work. According to Mme Rees, he was so poor at his job in electrical repairs that he was made archivist of his factory and finally given professional recognition by being elected a member of the Academy of the People's Republic of Romania (date unknown). He died in 1988. Valérie, a gynaecologist, visited the Rees family in England in 1989–90. Their son, Radu Serban Pascal, a junior tennis champion, became a political journalist, but fell out of favour after the 1989 revolution. He died in 1996 without children, which marks the end of the Pascal line in Romania.[15] Mme Rees also made contact with General Mengin's remaining relatives, none of whom had had any previous idea of her existence, or of this chapter in their family history. In 1974, she wrote to the Mayor of Colmy, a village near the Belgian border, asking for information about her father's family. The mayor put her in touch with the Génys, descendants of Mengin's sister's husband, who welcomed Jeanne and her husband. The families have remained in touch.[16]

15 For the shifts in Romanian allegiances during World War II see Evans, *Third Reich at War*, 618 and 653.

16 IJPR, 15–16 July 2002.

In the course of an active life, Jeanne Pascal Rees was determined to learn as much about her family origins as she could, to help those who had fallen on hard times after the war, to keep her mother's memory alive, to conserve the family archive and to become her mother's historian. It was not until 2001 in her article, 'À Propos de Constance Pascal', that she felt able to mention her own blood relationship with her mother and then without mentioning General Mengin by name, citing as her reason the respect she felt should be accorded to her parents' discretion under the pressure of the laws and prejudices of the time.

It has taken some fifty years for historians to explore Pascal's remarkable life and career, beginning with Jean-Michel Barbier's ground-breaking doctoral dissertation in 1989. As I have indicated, Pascal forbade any eulogies from her contemporaries. Brief official recognition did come in a short obituary by Dr Jacques Vié, her colleague at Maison Blanche, with whom she collaborated on their final unfinished work, *Hébéphrénie et terrain: mémoire pour la fondation de l'hébéphrénie* [Hebephrenia and its terrain: fundamental concepts: report on the underlying causes of hebephrenia].[17] Vié was a pioneer in the movement for *asiles de famille*, on the pattern of Geel in Belgium.[18] After serving at Charité sur Loire, Maison Blanche and Moisselles, he helped establish the Family Asylum of Ainey le Château. He was close to Constance Pascal, who wrote a dedication in his copy of *Chagrins d'Amour et psychoses*: 'À mon excellent collaborateur, Dr Vié, un témoignage de ma grande affection, Dr Pascal' [To my esteemed collaborator, Dr Vié, a testimony of my great affection, Dr Pascal]. He kept in touch with Jeanne after her mother's death.[19] Vié's first draft for an obituary of Pascal, which survives in longhand, is a more fitting and moving tribute to his friend and colleague than the drastically curtailed printed version:

> Mademoiselle C. Pascal: 1877–1937
>
> Une longue et douloureuse maladie vient d'emporter Mademoiselle le Docteur C. Pascal, médecin-chef de l'Hôpital psychiatrique de Maison Blanche à Neuilly sur Marne. Depuis près de 40 ans, sa vie était tout entière consacrée au traitement des malades mentaux et à la recherche scientifique dans le domaine si ardu de la psychiatrie.

17 Jacques Vié, 'Mademoiselle C. Pascal (1977–1937)', *La Presse médicale* (January 1938), 150. I am grateful to Margaret Rees for help in translation.

18 From medieval times, the town of Geel, pioneered the deinstitutionalization in psychiatric care by instituting family placements for mental patients. By 1938, over three and a half thousand patients were lodged with families in the town.

19 Interview with Mlle Vié, 27 March 2003.

Elle avait été jadis, en 1908, la première femme admise au concours de médecin des Asiles, et en 1925, elle devait, encore la première, franchir les barrières du concours spécial pour les asiles du département de la Seine.

Après avoir dans ses premiers travaux, pris pour guides les lois rigoureuses, mais statiques, de l'anatomie pathologique, Mlle Pascal avait dirigé, sous l'influence de son maître, M. Sérieux, la majeure partie de son labeur à l'une des maladies les plus redoutables et les plus mystérieuses, la démence précoce, qui, de jeunes gens parfois fort bien doués, fait en quelques mois de vrais déments, ou les réduit à n'être plus que des épaves sociales, de pauvres caricatures humaines, sans forces et sans désirs.

Mlle Pascal a pu arracher à ce fléau quelques bribes de son secret, elle en a précisé les symptômes d'alarme, les signes fondamentaux qui se cachent sous des aspects divers, le terrain sur lequel il se développe; à l'aide de tests pharmacodynamiques d'une grande délicatesse, elle a exploré les restes d'activité physique et mentale que cache le voile de la démence.

Jamais en effet elle n'avait oublié le but suprême de la médecine, réveiller ce qui subsiste encore, chez le malade, de vivant et de normal. Sans se décourager, elle a multiplié les essais thérapeutiques, mettant en œuvre les conquêtes les plus modernes de la biologie, notamment les traitements de choc, qui apportent des résultats parfois inespérés. Enfin elle développait toutes les modalités du traitement moral, montrant les multiples ressources qu'apporte auprès des malades – atteints non seulement dans l'esprit, mais bien souvent dans le cœur – la science animée par la sollicitude de l'affectivité féminine.

À l'asile de Châlons sur Marne, surmontant les nombreux obstacles que rencontrent les précurseurs, Mlle Pascal fondait et dirigeait, dès 1922, le premier institut consacré en province aux enfants anormaux.

Dans la Seine, elle se trouvait aux prises avec les innombrables problèmes médico-sociaux posés tous les jours à nos invalides du cerveau, si vulnérables par le surmenage de la grande ville, par la lutte pour la vie, trop âpre pour eux; elle se penchait sur les douloureux problèmes psychologiques des blessés du sentiment auxquels elle consacrait son dernier ouvrage, *Chagrins d'amour et psychoses*. Ainsi, Mlle Pascal n'avait jamais cessé d'être femme, et indépendamment d'une œuvre scientifique féconde, elle nous laisse une grande démonstration de féminisme en action: ce que peut réaliser, dans un domaine ardu comme celui des maladies mentales, l'alliance de l'intelligence et du cœur, sous la direction d'une courageuse indépendance de pensée scientifique.[20]

20 Jacques Vié, 'Obituary: Mademoiselle C. Pascal, Médecin en chef des Hôpitaux Psychiatriques de la Seine. 1877–1937' [Handwritten MS, unsigned, handwriting attested to by Dr Michel Caire].

[Dr Constance Pascal, 1877–1937

Dr Constance Pascal, *médecin-chef* at the Maison Blanche psychiatric hospital in Neuilly sur Marne, has just died after a long and painful illness. For almost forty years her life was wholly devoted to the treatment of the mentally ill and to scientific research in the taxing field of psychiatry.

Back in 1908, she was the first woman admitted to the examination for mental health specialists, and again in 1925 she was the first to break through the barrier of the special competitive examination for asylums of the Seine region.

In her earliest publications, Dr Pascal espoused the rigorous but rigid laws of pathological anatomy but later, under the influence of her supervisor Dr Sérieux, she focused the greater part of her research on one of the most frightful and mysterious illnesses, *dementia praecox*.[21] This condition has the power to turn young people, often the most gifted, in just a few months into truly demented creatures, or reduce them to social wrecks, pitiful caricatures without strength or motive. Dr Pascal forced this plague to yield just a few of its secrets: she specified its precipitating symptoms and essential signs, which may hide under a whole variety of appearances; she detailed the course of its development; and, by means of pharmacodynamic tests of great subtlety, she examined the last elements of physical and mental activity that survive behind the veil of madness.

Indeed, she never lost sight of the supreme aim of medicine: to reawaken whatever still remains alive and normal in the patient. Without losing heart, she multiplied her therapeutic efforts, exploiting the newest discoveries of biology, for example shock treatments, which sometimes produced unexpected successes. Finally, she employed all manner of psychological treatments, demonstrating just what can be done for patients – who often suffer not only in their minds but also in their hearts – by a combination of scientific knowledge with the tender care of womanly feeling.

At the Asylum of Châlons sur Marne, overcoming the many obstacles that stand in the way of any pioneer, Dr Pascal founded and directed, from 1922, the first provincial institute dedicated to the care of handicapped children.

Working in the Seine region, she found herself grappling with the many everyday medical and social problems of mental patients who fall victim to overwork or the stresses of urban existence, or who struggle to survive in the urban jungle; she concentrated in particular on the psychological problems of people suffering in their emotional lives, and devoted to them her last study, *Chagrins d'amour et psychoses*. As this suggests, Dr Pascal never ceased to be a woman and, quite

21 I am grateful to Dr Peter Eckstein for help with the medical vocabulary of this translation.

> independently of her prolific scientific production, she leaves to those who come after her an exceptional example of feminism in action, of what can be achieved, in a difficult field like that of mental illness, the union of the intelligence and the heart, overseen by a courageous mind schooled in the objectivity of scientific thought.]

Like the many journalists who had interviewed Pascal over the years, Vié praised her 'womanly' qualities, by which he may partly have meant that she represented the maternal ethos and thus, by eliding the gap between public and private, helped render women in the public sphere acceptable in the culture of the Third Republic.[22] Nevertheless, for Pascal's contemporaries, she also represented the embodiment of active feminism. Vié recognized too that in her passion for research, Pascal never lost her feeling for her patients as individuals, seeking to understand them in their milieu and to appreciate the accidents of life that had driven them to madness. There, but for her intellect and extraordinary willpower, she may have thought, she too might have gone. In her patients she recognized persons who had succumbed to unbearable conflicts or disappointments, not dissimilar to her own, but which, in her own case, she had succeeded in controlling and turning to good use in her profession.

Pascal's initial psychiatric training in pathological anatomy rested, in Vié's words, on assumptions about heredity as the principal factor in mental illness – the degeneration model. The fatalistic assumptions behind this model were ones that she increasingly contested in the course of her career. In the 1920s she enthusiastically participated in the therapeutic impulse, characterized by experiments in shock therapy and efforts to understand the biological bases of madness, for this allowed for a more active and hopeful confrontation with the scourge of mental illness. Finally, and most significantly perhaps, her growing recognition of the social factors underlying the conditions of her women patients at Maison Blanche pointed to a radical analysis of gender construction. These were women on whom the sorrows of love weighed disproportionately, in that their sense of self-worth was entirely determined by their ability to be loved. Her views on the inevitable disappointments of love in *Chagrins d'amour et psychoses*, no doubt reflect her own experience, but also, more profoundly, the destabilising effect for women of linking their entire destiny to some

22 For the ethos of maternalism as eliding the gap between the public and private spheres in the Third republic see Elinor A. Accampo, Rachel G. Fuchs and Mary Lynn Stewart, *Gender and the Politics of Social Reform in France 1870–1914* (Baltimore and London: Johns Hopkins University Press, 1995), 1–27.

version of romantic love.[23] One can argue that Pascal's profession liberated her from the cul-de-sac of frustrated or disappointed love, which she might have recognized, in her admiration for Freud, as creative sublimation. She poured her emotional energy into her psychiatric work. This was, as Vié noted, feminism in action, proving by example that a woman need not be defined entirely by her biology, or by the gender expectations of her age.

One of the most compelling aspects of Pascal's character and career rests on the disjunction between her professional and private lives, a disjunction imposed by a combination of factors: her own background, her dedication to her profession, her emotional disappointments, her devotion to her daughter and the social milieu in which she lived. Having chosen to keep her child, she was haunted, nevertheless, by the hypocrisy she felt forced to practise. She made it a labour of love to prepare Jeanne to fit a society in which her illegitimate status could well have compromised her chances of happiness or success. Yet for Pascal, as for her patient who had been 'cured by joy', motherhood, whatever its risks and drawbacks, 'ouvrit les portes du paradis' (JPR, Mémoires, 184) [opened the gates of paradise].

To estimate Pascal's qualities and the effect she had on her contemporaries is not easy. Observers speak of her authoritative presence and dignity. She was intellectually brilliant, proud and, as a young woman, very beautiful. Superbly educated in the arts and humanities as well as in the sciences, she spoke at least five languages. Throughout her life she read widely in literature, history and philosophy. Though she had great charm when she chose to exercise it, she could be acerbic when confronted with what she considered stupidity or masculine pomposity, and chafed under the weight of organizational torpor in many of the asylums where she worked. She was a thorn in the side of civil servants and hospital administrators. Though often desperately unhappy and self-pitying, she possessed a counterbalancing sense of irony. Her political sympathies, broadly on the left, were combined with strong anticlericalism, another mark of the French professional elite of that period. As her friend Mathilde Salomon had said when Pascal first qualified in psychiatry, she was a feminist by example rather than by public agitation.[24] She was an intellectual elitist who worked all her professional life with society's most marginalized individuals. Internally she was wracked by anger, loneliness and guilt, yet she demonstrated a moving capacity for love in her care and concern for her daughter, and showed a generosity of

23 *CAP*, 165–67.

24 Corr CP & MS, PRFP February 1909.

spirit towards General Mengin, albeit coupled with a certain disdain. Her commitment to psychiatric research continued until her death. She found her patients, whom she loved, endlessly fascinating.

Pascal died before Hitler's war and would have been devastated to see her native country fighting in alliance with Germany. During the First World War, before Romania opted for the Allies, she had agonized in her journal about which side it would choose. Her admiration and love for France is one of the major themes of those years. France's defeat, its capitulation to Germany and the establishment of the Vichy regime in 1940 would have horrified her.[25] In any case, she would have been disqualified from continuing in her profession by the law of 17 July 1940, promulgated by Marshall Pétain. This decreed that no one could be employed in public service without possessing French nationality, which could only be derived from a French-born father.[26] Pascal's naturalization as a French citizen would have counted for nothing. It would have been worse, perhaps, to continue working in psychiatric hospitals during the prolonged Vichy food rationing that deprived many patients, especially the elderly, of sufficient nourishment to support life. Pascal's Maison Blanche succumbed, like other psychiatric hospitals, to starving its patients, not by design but because the official food rations were totally insufficient:

> L'hôpital vit dans cette période de restrictions un terrible drame, comme la quasi-totalité des hôpitaux psychiatriques français. […] Le taux de mortalité annuel, qui était à Maison Blanche de 9% avant l'Occupation, passe à plus de 14% en 1940, plus de 28% en 1941, et 29.35% en 1942. On compte, en 1941, 694 décès de tuberculose, mais aussi et surtout de faim.[27]
>
> [In that period of restrictions, the hospital witnessed a terrible tragedy, like almost all the psychiatric hospitals in France. […] The annual death rate, which was 9% at Maison Blanche before the Occupation, rose to over 14% in 1940, over 28% in 1941 and 29.35% in 1942. In 1941, 694 are said to have died – many of tuberculosis, but also, above all, of hunger.]

There was no great epidemic to account for these mortality figures, except an epidemic of starvation. In asylums throughout France,

25 On the French defeat and capitulation and German triumph see Evans, *The Third Reich at War*, 131–33.

26 Linda L. Clark, *The Rise of Professional Women in France*, 244.

27 Michel Caire, 'Maison Blanche sous l'Occupation', *Maison Blanche: le centenaire*, 69.

death mowed down thousands of skeletal men and women, huddled in dark, dirty and unheated wards. At Maison Blanche, the patients employed to peel vegetables ate them uncooked. Those who enjoyed a little freedom to roam the grounds gathered mushrooms by the kilo on the hospital lawns and ate them raw. Some ate grass in the courtyards.[28] Although food restrictions applied throughout French society, people in the wider community at least had the possibility of finding food supplements either in the black market, by barter, or by growing their own. But rations in the hospitals were strictly limited and closely supervised and with few exceptions hospital authorities were unable or unwilling to attempt extra-legal methods of acquiring more food for the patients. Had Pascal witnessed this human disaster in which the most vulnerable in society, to whom she had devoted her career, were considered expendable, or at least not worthy of efforts to save them, she might well have felt that her life's work counted for nothing. In 1952, Georges Daumézon who, as a young man, had asked Pascal for advice on pursuing a career in psychiatry, looked back despairingly on the Vichy period, writing: 'De 1940 à 1944 nous, Français, nous avons laissé mourir de faim 40,000 aliénés' [From 1940 to 1944, we, the French, allowed 40,000 mental patients to die of hunger].[29]

This holocaust of the mad, to cite Isabelle von Bueltzingsloewen's 2007 title, made crystal clear the weaknesses of the old psychiatric regime of incarcerating large numbers of mental patients in huge hospitals. Under Vichy they became hostages to famine. The post-war reaction against the massification of asylum culture and movement towards a system of out-patient clinics and open-door policies in psychiatric hospitals, while general across Europe, was in France part of a painful reckoning with the years of the Occupation. In the previous generation, these changes had been foreshadowed by the work of Édouard Toulouse, Jacques Vié and Constance Pascal, as well as many other psychiatric reformers.[30] Nevertheless, in defending the law of 1838 (which created the public asylums) because she believed

28 Michel Caire, 'Maison Blanche sous l'Occupation', 70. See also Bueltzingsloeven, *L'Hécatombe des fous*.

29 Georges Daumézon, 'Le poids des structures', *Esprit* (1952), 943, quoted in Michel Caire, 'Un établissement du dispositif de la Seine: l'hôpital psychiatrique de Maison-Blanche', *Morts d'inanition: Famine et exclusions en France sous l'Occupation*, ed. by Isabelle von Bueltzingsloewen (Rennes: Presses Universitaires de Rennes, 2005), 108.

30 Nicolas Henckes, 'Réformer et soigner: l'émergence de la psychothérapie institutionnelle en France, 1944–1955, *Psychiatries dans l'histoire* (Caen: PUC, 2008), 277–88.

it protected vulnerable psychiatric patients, Pascal was, like so many of her colleagues, arguably a part of the problem as well as working toward its solution.[31] Her work encompasses the strengths, the creative energies and the weaknesses of the French asylum system. Within the constraints of that institutional framework, Pascal showed herself to be innovative, compassionate and reforming. Given her status as a female 'first' in psychiatry, a status that she found somewhat wearisome by the end of her career, her patient-centred therapeutic methods were interpreted as evidence of a maternal ethos. An intellectual, a woman who felt bitterly about the constraints on her own girlhood, a psychiatrist devoted to attempting to heal the mad, Constance Pascal remains an iconic figure who can move us by her passion for her profession, her love for her daughter and her sense of loss, anger and misery at the social pressures under which she laboured, many of which she recognized as afflicting her female patients.

In his re-publication of Pascal's *Chagrins d'amour et psychoses* in 2000, sixty-five years after its first publication, Jacques Chazaud paid generous tribute on behalf of historians of psychiatry to Pascal's work as a clinician, to her innovative educational schemes for children with severe learning difficulties and to her interest in developing open psychiatric clinics and encouraging psychotherapy in the treatment of asylum patients.[32] Nevertheless, the originality of her contributions was forgotten for over half a century, partly by her own wish and partly by the repudiation by the post-war generation of psychiatrists of previous asylum policies following the catastrophic loss of life in psychiatric hospitals under Vichy. Even a recent historical re-evaluation which pays tribute to the reforming efforts of Georges Dauмézon, a psychiatrist who, as we have seen, took his inspiration from Pascal, 'la Grande Dame de la medicine mentale' [the *grande dame* of mental medicine], overlooks her work.[33] It is important to reintegrate Constance Pascal fully both into the history of psychiatry, as Jean-Michel Barbier, Jacques Chazaud, Michel Caire and Jeanne Pascal Rees have all helped to do, and into the broader perspective of women's and feminist history, in order to commemorate and understand her achievements. She was, in Michel Caire's words: 'incontestablement l'une des plus dynamiques et des plus modernes des aliénistes de son temps' (Caire, 'Constance Pascal',

31 Pascal, 'Les Asiles ne sont pas des geôles'.

32 Jacques Chazaud, 'Avant-propos éditorial', Constance Pascal, *Chagrins d'amour et psychoses*, ii–v.

33 Chazaud, 'Avant propos', ii; Henckes, 'Réformer', 277–88.

7) [indisputably one of the most dynamic and advanced psychiatrists of her time].

The personal conflicts of her private life, disguised by her assured though sometimes highly emotional and combative performance in the public arena, are symptomatic of the costs and rewards for the women of her generation, who entered and rose in the professions. Pascal forged her multiple roles into an authoritative and compassionate identity that marks her as a woman for whom a burning ambition for professional success remained focused on the care of others marked by 'un attachement fait d'intelligente pitié [affection based on intelligent pity].[34] From patients with *dementia praecox* to the psychotic women in her wards at Maison Blanche, from the epileptics incarcerated at that time in mental hospitals to the children and adults with severe learning difficulties, Pascal took on a constituency of the afflicted who could not speak for themselves. Yet it was not only compassion that motivated her, but also her delight in the complexity of the human mind. She represented, as her nephew Ion Pascal wrote: 'un idéal, la passion du travail, la forme la plus noble de l'ambition qui ne trouve son apaisement que dans le travail désintéressé' (Corr JP & JP, Berlin, PRFP 13 May 1938) [an ideal, the passion for work, the noblest form of ambition that only finds its satisfaction in disinterested labour]. As a woman in a profession which, at her death, was still dominated by men, she became a symbol of feminist aspirations. She demonstrated, by the rigour and breadth of her intellect and what Vié termed; 'l'alliance de l'intelligence et du cœur' [the union of the intelligence and the heart], her humane commitment to her patients and the capacity of women to succeed in the most arduous of callings.

34 L. M. Compain, 'Une femme médecin d'un asile d'aliénés', *La Petite République* (1911).

Bibliography

Archival Sources

Archives Historiques de la Ministère de Défense, Armée de la Terre, Vincennes, Dossier Justin Mengin, Gyd 604 Mengin

Archives de la Marne

Archives Nationales Fontainebleau, Centre d'Archives Contemporaines, 19810706 art/ 14, Dossier Pascal, 1908–1930

Archives de la Ville de Paris VK2 2108, Dossier administratif, Maison Blanche, Constance Pascal

Archives de la Ville de Paris, Série D1 K1 0424, Bulletin des lois de la république française XIIe série – note of Constance Pascal's naturalisation

Archives de la Ville de Paris, Commission de Surveillances des Asiles Publics d'Aliénés du Département de la Seine

Bibliothèque Marguerite Durand

Centre Hospitalier de Clermont de l'Oise: Dossier Administratif Constance Pascal

Centre Hospitalier de Maison Blanche: Dossier Administratif Constance Pascal

Centre Hospitalier de Moisselles: Dossier Administratif Constance Pascal

Centre Hospitalier de Prémontré: Dossier Administratif Constance Pascal

Communication from Margaret Rees, 13 April 2003

Fonds Marie Louise Bouglé, Bibliothèque Historique de la Ville de Paris

Interviews with Jeanne Pascal Rees, 19 March 2002, 15–16 July 2002, 24 October 2002, 20 November 2002, 17 June 2003

Mémoires Jeanne Pascal Rees

Pascal/Rees Family Papers
Rapports sur les Asiles d'Aliénés du Département de la Seine: Centre Hospitalier de Moisselles
Rapports sur les Asiles d'Aliénés du Département de la Seine: Centre Hospitalier de Maison Blanche
Rapports de Mlle le Dr C. Pascal, 1925–26, Archives Nationales, Centre des Archives Contemporaines de Fontainebleau
Rapports de Mlle le Dr C. Pascal, 1927–35, Archives Nationales, Centre des Archives Contemporaines de Fontainebleau

Printed Sources

Abir-Am, Pnina G. and Dorinda Outram (eds.) *Uneasy Careers and Intimate Lives: Women in Science 1789–1979* (New Brunswick and London: Rutgers University Press, 1989)
Accampo, Elinor A., 'Private life, public image: motherhood and militancy in the self-construction of Nelly Roussel, 1900–1922', in Jo Burr Margadant (ed.), *The New Biography: Performing Femininity in Nineteenth-Century France* (Berkeley, Los Angeles and London: University of California Press, 2000), 172–218
Accampo, Elinor A., Rachel G. Fuchs and Mary Lynn Stewart, *Gender and the Politics of Social Reform in France 1870–1914* (Baltimore and London: Johns Hopkins University Press, 1995)
'Actes de la journée du centenaire de Maison Blanche 22 juin 2000', *Maison Blanche, centenaire 1900–2000.* Établissement public de santé Maison Blanche
Adreani, A., *La Condition des étrangers en France et la législation sur la nationalité française* (Paris: Librairie Guillaumin et Cie, 1896)
Allard, Paul, 'Folles d'amour: heures dans un asile', *Vu* (1933), PRFP
Anon., 'Les Femmes internes dans les asiles de la Seine', *La Fronde* (1 Jan, 1904), BMD
— 'Femmes internes, hôpitaux et asiles', *La Vie Heureuse* (Feb. 1905a), BMD
— 'Une nouvelle doctoresse', *La Fronde* (8 Juin, 1905b), BMD
— 'La doctoresse Pascal à l'asile de Ville Evrard', periodical unknown (1905c), PRFP
— Journal de la Marne (August ? 1925), PRFP
— 'Woman of the day', *Paris Times*, no. 325 (1925), PRFP

Barbier, Jean-Michel, 'La vie et l'œuvre de Constance Pascal (1877–1937)', Thèse pour le Doctorat en Médecine, Diplôme d'État (Université de Picardie: Faculté de Médicine d'Amiens, 9 Janvier, 1997)

Barbier, Jean-Michel, Gérard Serra and Gwenolé Loas, 'Constance Pascal: pioneer of French psychiatry', *History of Psychiatry* 10 (1999), 425–37

Bard, Christine, *Madeleine Pelletier: Logique et infortunes d'un combat pour l'égalité* (Paris: Côté Femmes, 1992)

— *Les Garçonnes: modes et fantasmes des années folles* (Paris: Flammarion, 1998)

— *Les Femmes dans la société française au 20e siècle* (Paris: Armand Colin, 2001)

Barnel, F., 'Madeleine Pelletier, 1874–1939: première femme interne des asiles de la Seine', Thèse d'État, Médecine (Paris VI: Université Pierre et Marie Curie, 1988)

Baruk, Henri, *La Psychiatrie française de Pinel à nos jours* (Paris: PUF, 1967)

Basch, Victor, *Schumann: A Life of Suffering*, trans. by C.A. Phillips (New York: Alfred A. Knopf, 1936); originally published in French, 1928

Becker, Annette, *Oubliés de la Grand Guerre* (Paris: Éditions Noêsis, 1998)

Bécoulet, Dr, 'Étude sur Le No-Restraint', *Annales médico-psychologiques*, 6e série, 4e année, VII (Paris: Masson, 1882), 41–69

Bell, Susan Groag, and Karen M. Offen (eds.) *Women, the Family and Freedom* (Stanford, CA: Stanford University Press, 1983)

Bellanger, Claude, Jacques Godechot, Pierre Guiral and François Terrou, *Histoire générale de la presse française; Tome II De 1871–1940* (Paris: Presses Universitaires de France, 1972)

Berger-Leuvrault, Oscar, *Dictionnaire militaire* (Paris: Alcan, 1910)

Bergson, Henri, *Essai sur les données immédiates de la conscience* (Paris: Alcan, 1901)

Binet, Alfred, 'Ribot et la psychologie scientifique française', *Centenaire de Th. Ribot: jubilé de la psychologie scientifique française 1839–1889–1939* (Agen: Imprimerie Moderne, 1939), 109–13

Blancpain, Marc, *La Vie quotidienne dans la France du nord sous les occupations 1814–1944* (Paris: Hachette, 1983)

Bleuler, Eugen, *Dementia Praecox: oder Gruppe der Schizophrenien* (Leipzig: F. Deuticke, 1911)

Boissel, Anne, 'Les enfants de Caïn, Louis Roubaud', *La Lettre de l'enfance et de l'adolescence* 1, 2006 (n° 63), 7–10, www.cairn.info/revue-lettre-de-l-enfance-et-de-l-adolescence-2006–1–page-7.htm [acessed 19 September 2012]

Bonner, Thomas N., *To the Ends of the Earth: Women's Search for Education in Medicine* (Cambridge, MA and London: Harvard University Press, 1992)

Bonvoisin, Samra-Martine and Michèle Maignien, *La Presse féminine* (Paris: Presses Universitaires de France, 1986)

Bourget, Paul, *La Geôle* (Paris: Plon, 1923)

Bradamante, 'Le mariage des officiers', *La Fronde* (28 December 1921)

Butler, Judith, 'Performative acts and gender construction: an essay in phenomenology and feminist theory', in Sue-Ellen Case (ed.), *Performing Feminisms: Feminist Critical Theory and Theatre* (Baltimore and London: John Hopkins University Press, 1990)

von Bueltzingsloewen, Isabelle, *Morts d'inanition: famine et exclusions en France sous l'Occupation* (Rennes: Presses Universitaires de Rennes, 2005)

— *L'Hécatombe des fous: la famine dans les hôpitaux psychiatriques français sous l'Occupation* (Paris: Aubier, 2007)

Buvat-Pochon, Christine, *Les Traitements de choc d'autrefois en psychiatrie* (Paris: Librairie le François, 1939)

Caire, Michel, 'Constance Pascal', http://psychiatrie.histoire.free.fr/pers/bio/pascal.htm (2007) [accessed 19 September 2012]

Capgras, Joseph, 'Réformes de déments précoces', *Annales médico-psychologiques* II (1918), 111–23

Castel, Robert, *L'Ordre psychiatrique: l'âge d'or de l'aliénisme* (Paris: Editions Minuit, 1976)

Charle, Christophe, *Le Siècle de la presse: 1830–1939* (Paris: Seuil, 2004)

Charpentier, Joseph. 'Un asile martyre, Prémontré pendant la guerre', *L'Informateur des aliénistes,* 16e année, 1 (25 January 1921), 154–59

Charpentier, R., Announcement of C. Pascal's death, *Société Médico Psychologique* (25 December 1937)

Charrier, Edmée, *L'Évolution intellectuelle féminine* (Paris: Librairie du Recueil Sirey, 1937)

Chazaud, Jacques, 'Constance Pascal, première femme aliéniste en France', *Histoire des sciences médicales* XXV 1 (2001), 85–90

Christian, J., 'De la démence précoce des jeunes gens', *Annales médico-psychologiques,* Tome IX (March-April 1899), 43–69, 200–16, (May–June 1899), 420–32, Tome X (September – October 1899), 177–88

Clark, Linda. L., *The Rise of Professional Women in France: Gender and Public Administration since 1830* (Cambridge: Cambridge University Press, 2000)

— *Women and Achievement in Nineteenth-Century Europe* (Cambridge: Cambridge University Press, 2008)

Clout, Hugh D, 'Rural revival in the Marne, 1914–1930', *Agricultural Historical Review*, 42, II (1993), 140–55

Compain, L.-M., 'Une femme médecin d'un asile d'aliénés', *La Petite République* (1911), Clermont DACP

Corradi, Consuelo, 'Text, context and individual meaning: rethinking life stories in a hermeneutic framework', *Discourse and Society* 2 (1), (1991), 105–18

Courbon, unpublished ms. Courtesy of Dr. Jacques Chazaud, PRFP

Creese, Mary R.S., *Ladies in the Laboratory II: West European Women in Science, 1800–1900* (Lanham, MD and Oxford: The Scarecrow Press, 2004)

Croubois, Claude, *L'Officier français des origines à nos jours* (Saint-Jean-d'Angely: Editions Bordessoules, 1987)

Dalloz, Désiré, 'Mariage', *Nouveau Répertoire de Droit*, III (Paris: Dalloz, 1964), 257–62

Dalloz, Armand, *Recueil périodique et critique* (Paris: Dalloz, 1923)

Demay, G., Review: '*Chagrins d'amour et psychoses*, par le Docteur Constance Pascal', *L'Aliéniste français: bulletin de l'association amicale des médecins des établissements publics d'aliénés* (July 1935), 414–15

Dowbiggin, Ian R., *Inheriting Madness: Professionalization and Psychiatric Knowledge in Nineteenth-Century France* (Berkeley and Oxford: University of California Press, 1991)

Duby, Georges and Michelle Perrot, *Histoire des femmes: le XIXe siècle* (Paris: Plon, 1991)

Duché Didier, Jacques, *Histoire de la psychiatrie de l'enfant* (Paris: Presses Universitaires de France, 1990)

Durandin, Catherine, *Histoire des roumains* (Paris: Fayard, 1995)

Duroselle, Jean-Baptiste, *La Grande Guerre des français* (Paris: Perrin, 1995)

Émile-Magne, Élise, 'La première femme aliéniste de la Seine', *La Française* (1925), PRFP

Evans, Richard J., *The Feminists* (London & Sydney: Croom Helm, 1977)

— *In Defence of History* (London: Granta Books, 1997)

— *The Third Reich at War: How the Nazis led Germany from conquest to disaster* (London: Allen Lane, 2008)

— 'The Tory interpretation of history', *London Review of Books* 33 (6) (17 March 2011), 9–12

Fauvel, Annette, 'Le crime de Clermont et la remise en cause des asiles en 1880', *Revue d'histoire moderne et contemporaine* (2002), 49–61

— 'Punition, dégénérescence ou malheur? La folie d'André Gill (1840–1885)', *Revue d'histoire du XIXe siècle* (2003), 26–27

Fee, Elizabeth, 'Nineteenth-century craniology: the study of the female skull', *Bulletin of the History of Medicine*, 53 (1979), 423–33

Fink, Max, 'Induced seizures and human behaviour', Max Fink, S. Kety, J. McGaugle and T. Williams (eds.), *Psychobiology of Convulsive Therapy* (Washington D.C.: V. H. Winston, 1974)

— 'Meduna and the origins of convulsive therapy', *American Journal of Psychiatry* (1984), 1034–1041

— *Electroshock: Healing and Mental Illness* (Oxford: Oxford University Press, 2002)

Foucault, André, 'Les acuités sensorielles et les enfants arriérés ou retardés', *Journal de psychologie normale et pathologique* (1924), 219–35

Foucault, Michel, *La Folie et la déraison: histoire de la folie à l'âge classique* (Paris: Plon, 1961)

— *Surveiller et punir, naissance de la prison* (Paris: Gallimard, 1975)

Frizot, Michel. 'Looking at Vu : a photographic magazine; 1928–1940', www.mep-fr.org/us/actu/vu.htm [accessed 19 September 2012]

Fuchs, Rachel G, *Contested Paternity: Constructing Families in Modern France* (Baltimore: John Hopkins University Press, 2008)

Gaillac, Henri, *Les Maisons de correction 1830–1945* (Paris: Éditions Cujas, 1971)

Gaines, Ruth, *A Village in Picardie* (New York: E.P. Dutton, 1918)

Gilberg, Trond, 'The multiple legacies of history: Romania in the year 1990' in Joseph Held (ed.), *The Columbia History of Eastern Europe in the Twentieth Century* (New York: Columbia University Press, 1991)

Giroud, Françoise, *Une Femme honorable* (Paris: Fayard, 1981)

Goldstein, Jan, *Console and Classify: The French Psychiatric Profession in the Nineteenth Century* (Cambridge: Cambridge University Press, 1987)

Gordon, Felicia, *The Integral Feminist: Madeleine Pelletier, 1874–1939* (Cambridge: Polity Press, 1990)

— 'French psychiatry and the new woman: the case of Dr Constance Pascal, 1877–1937', *History of Psychiatry* 17 (2) (2006), 159–82

— 'Publicity and professionalism: Madeleine Pelletier (1874–1939) and Constance Pascal (1877–1937)', *Modern and Contemporary France* 17 (3) (2009), 319–34

— 'Women in French medicine and psychiatry in the *Belle Époque*: a feminist cause?', *Maturitas* 68 (2011), 268–71

Gould, Stephen Jay, *The Mismeasure of Man* (London: Norton, 1981)

Grogan, Susan K., *French Socialism and Sexual Difference: Women and the New Society, 1803–44* (Basingstoke: Macmillan, 1992)

Henckes, Nicolas, 'Réformer et soigner: l'émergence de la psychothérapie institutionnelle en France, 1944–1955, *Psychiatries dans l'histoire* (Caen: Presses Universitaires de Caen, 2008), 277–88

Heuyer, Georges, *Enfants anormaux et délinquants juvéniles* (Paris: G. Steenheil, 1914)

— *Le Niveau intellectuel des enfants d'âge scolaire, travaux et documents, cahier 13* (Paris: Presses Universitaires Françaises, 1950)

Horne, Alistair, *The French Army and Politics: 1870–1970* (London: Macmillan, 1984)

Hunt, Neil, *Bipolar Disorder: Your Questions Answered* (Edinburgh: Elsevier, 2005)

Huteau, Michel, *Psychologie, psychiatrie et société sous la Troisième République: la biocratie d'Édouard Toulouse, 1865–1947* (Paris: L'Harmattan, 2002)

Joël, Constance, *Les Filles d'Esculape* (Paris: Édition Robert Laffont, 1988)

Jolly, Jean, 'Paul Strauss: ancien sénateur de la Seine', *Dictionnaire des parlementaires français* (Paris: Presses Universitaires de France, 1960–1977)

Jordan, Jack, 'The Unconscious', in Richard Bales (ed.), *The Cambridge Companion to Proust* (Cambridge: Cambridge University Press, 2001).

Kadar, Marlene, *Essays on Life Writing* (Toronto and London: University of Toronto Press, 1992)

Kraepelin, Emil, *Dementia Praecox and Paraphrenia,* trans. by R. Mary Barclay from the 8th German edition, ed. by George M. Robertson (Edinburgh: Livingstone, 1919)

Klippel and J. Lhermitte, 'Les démences, anatomie, pathologie et pathogénie', *Revue de psychiatrie* (1905), 485–518

Kristeva, Julia, *Histoires d'amour* (Paris: Denvel, 1983)

Kuhn, Ronald, 'Eugen Bleuler's concepts of psychopathology', *History of Psychiatry,* 15 (3), 361–62

William L. Langer, *Encyclopaedia of World History* (Boston, Mass: Houghton Mifflin, 1952)

Lanteri-Laura, Georges, 'La place de la notion de schizophrénie dans la tradition psychiatrique française', *Synapse* (December 1988)

Leahey, Thomas. H., *A History of Psychology: Main Currents in Psychological Thought* (Upper Saddle River, NJ: Prentice Hall, 2000)

Lepinska, Mélanie, *Histoire des femmes médecins* (Paris: Librairie G. Jacques et Cie, 1900)

Lequin, Yves, *Histoire des étrangers et de l'immigration en France* (Paris: Larousse, 1992)

Loas, Gwenolé, 'News and notes', *History of Psychiatry VII* (1996), 341–42

Lombroso, Cesare, *L'Homme de génie* [L'huomo de genio in rapporto alla psichiatria] (1888), trans. Colonna d'Istria (Paris: Alcan, 1909)

Macintyre, Ben, *A Foreign Field* (London: Harper Collins, 2001)

McMillan, James F., *Housewife or Harlot, the Place of Women in French Society, 1870–1940* (Brighton: Harvester Press, 1981)

— *France and Women 1789–1914: Gender, Society and Politics* (London and New York: Routledge, 2000)

McPhail, Helen, *The Long Silence: Civilian Life Under the German Occupation of Northern France, 1914–1918* (London: I. B. Tauris, 1999)

Manouvrier, Léonce, 'Conclusions générales sur l'anthropologie des sexes et ses applications sociales', *Revue de l'École d'Anthropologie de Paris*, 13 (1903), 405–23

Margadant, Jo Burr, *Madame le Professeur: Women Educators in the Third Republic* (Princeton: Princeton University Press, 1990)

— *The New Biography: Performing Femininity in Nineteenth-Century France*, (Berkeley, CA and London: University of California Press, 2000)

— Review, 'Contested Paternity: Constructing Families in Modern France, *Journal of Social History* (1 July 2010)

Marston, Frank S., *The Peace Conference of 1919: Organization and Procedure* (London: and New York: Oxford University Press, 1944)

Mayeur, Françoise, *L'Enseignement secondaire des jeunes filles sous la Troisième République* (Paris: Presse de la Fondation Nationale des Sciences Politiques, 1977)

— *L'Éducation des filles en France au XIXe siècle* (Paris: Hachette, 1979)

— *Histoire générale de l'enseignement et de l'éducation en France de la révolution à l'école républicaine*, III (Paris: Nouvelle Librairie de France, 1981)

— 'Women and elites from the nineteenth to the twentieth century', in Loyon Howorth and Philip G. Cerny (eds.), *Elites in France: Origins, Reproduction and Power* (London: Frances Pinter, 1981)

Moll, Marie José and Jean-Claude Pėna, 'L'architecture asilaire, de 1900 à nos jours', *Maison Blanche le centenaire,* (2000), 37–43

Moote, Alanson Lloyd, 'New bottles and new wine: the current state of early modernist biographical writing', *French Historical Studies* 19 (4) (1996), 911–26

Morel, Bénédict, *Traité des maladies mentale,* 2nd ed. (Paris: Ballière, 1860)

Motte, de la, Dean, J. M. Przyblyski, *Modernity and the Mass Press in Nineteenth-Century France* (Amherst: University of Massachusetts, 1999)

Murat, Laure, *La Maison du Docteur Blanche* (Paris: Hachette, 2001)

Nicault, Catherine, 'Mathilde Salomon, pédagogue et pionnière de l'éducation féminine', *Archives juives* 1 (37) (2004)

Offen, Karen, *European Feminisms 1700–1950* (Stanford, CA: Stanford University Press, 2000)

Ogilvie, Marilyn B. & Joy Harvey (eds)., *The Biographical Dictionary of Women in Science: Pioneering Lives from Ancient Times to the Mid-Twentieth-Century* (New York and London: Routledge, 2000)

— *Marie Curie: a Biography* (Westport, CT and London: Greenwood Press, 2004)

Ohayon, Annick, *L'Impossible rencontre: psychologie et psychanalyse en France 1919–1969* (Paris: Éditions de la découverte, 1999)

Ostwald, Peter, *Schumann: Music and Madness* (London: Victor Gollancz, 1985)

Pascal, Constance, *Formes atypiques de la paralysie générale: prédominances régionales des lésions dans les méningo-encéphalites diffuses* (Paris: Thèse d'État: Médecine, 1905)

— 'Formes prodromiques dépressives de la démence précoce', *Informateur des aliénistes et des neurologistes* I (1906), 186–88

— 'Les ictus dans la démence précoce', *L'Encéphale* 1 (5) (25 September 1906), 139–44

— 'La loi roumaine sur les aliénés: traduction et réflexions', *Journal de médicine légale, psychiatrique et d'anthropologie criminelle* I (1906), 204–13

— 'Le sourire et le rire dans la démence précoce', *Journal de psychologie* 6 (1906), 392–407

— 'Formes mélancoliques dans la démence précoce', *Archives de neurologie* (April 1907), 273–93

— 'Les rémissions dans la démence précoce', *Revue de psychiatrie* (April 1907), 147–61

— 'Pseudo-neurasthénie prodromique de la démence précoce', *La Presse médicale* I (1907), 42–44

— 'Les maladies mentales de Robert Schumann', *Journal de psychologie normale et pathologique* 5 (1908), 98–130
— 'La démence précoce', *Revue de médecine* XXXI (1911), 304–33
— *La Démence précoce* (Paris: Librairie Félix Alcan, 1911)
— 'L'enfance anormale dans les maisons de correction', *Revue philanthropique* XXXIV (1913–14), 260–71
— 'Forme paranoïde de la paralysie générale', *L'Encéphale* 9 (6) (10 June 1914), 544–50
— 'La protection des enfants', *Le Petit écho de la mode* (25 March 1917), PRFP
— 'La femme française votera-t-elle?', *La Voix commune* (13 April 1919), PRFP
— 'La suppression des garderies de fous', *La Presse médicale* (September 1921), 1389–91
— 'Syndrome psychique fondamental des démences', *Journal de psychologie normale et pathologique* (1923), 146–56
— 'Les asiles d'aliénés ne sont pas des geôles', *Le Matin* (1924), PRFP
— 'Les grands syndromes psychiatriques: les démences', *Nouveau traité de médecine* (February 1927), 7–125
— 'Chagrins d'amour et psychoses', *Le Progrès médical* 36 (September 1932), 1513–1524
— *Le Dynamisme de la démence précoce* (Paris: Masson, 1932)
— 'Le brouillard étiologique de la démence précoce s'est-il dissipé?', *Le Progrès médicale,* 32 (1933), 1419–1435
— 'Réflexions sur le concours du médicat des asiles de 1933: pourquoi le médecin aliéniste doit être polyvalent?', MS (1933), PRFP
— *Chagrins d'amour et psychoses* (Paris: Doin & Cie, 1935), 2nd ed. (Paris: Harmattan, 2000)
— 'La pathologie des refuges', *Paris médical* (11 March 1936), 221–25
Pascal, Constance and Dr Courbon, 'Délire des préjudices préséniles', *L'Encéphale* 6 (25 Nov. 1906), 573–78
Pascal, Constance and Jean Davesne, *Anaphylaxie mentale spontanée* (Paris: Masson, 1925)
— 'La psychiatrie d'urgence'. *La Pratique médicale française* (1925), 458–68
— 'Les psychocolloïdoclasies: anaphylaxie mental spontanée', *La Presse médicale* (November 1925), 1539–41
— 'La thérapeutique sanguine dans les psychoses', *La Presse médicale* no. 67 (1925), 1126
— 'Les abcès de fixation dans les psychoses', *Archives internationales de neurologie* (1926), 41–55

— 'Chocs émotionnels pathogènes et thérapeutiques', *Journal de psychologie* 23 (1926), 456–87
— *Le Traitement des maladies mentales par les chocs* (Paris: Masson, 1926)
Pascal, Constance and F. Laurent, 'Abcès de fixation et examen du fond mental', *Annales médico-psychologiques* 12e série, tome II (1922), 320–29
Pascal, Constance, R. Abramovitz and M. Briau, 'Amélioration rapide d'une paralytique générale cachectique et gâteuse par le Stovarsol associée au Dmelcos (vaccin anti- chancrelleux de Nicolle)', *Annales médico-psychologiques* I (1928), 222–26
Pascal, Constance, Jacques Vié and Paul Agasse, 'Guérison rapide d'une influencée catatonique (démence paranoïde?) à la suite de vaccination anti typhique', *L'Encéphale* 23 (10) (December 1928), 937–40
— 'Impulsions homicides chez une mélancolique intermittente attente d'encéphalite', *L'Encéphale* 24 (1929), 361–422
Pascal, Constance and Jacques Vié, 'Étude critique des morphogrammes schizoïdes de Kretschmer', *Annales médico-psychologiques* I (1930), 154–63
— *Démence précoce et schizophrénie de Kretschmer Morel et la notion du terrain dans la démence précoce* (Paris: G. Doin, 1931)
Pascal, Constance and Andrée Deschamps, 'Psychoses de sensibilisation: allergie mentale', *Annales médico-psychologiques* I (May 1931), 449–60 and II (June 1931), 8–20
— *Exploration pharmacodynamique de la motricité des déments précoces* (Paris: G. Dolu, 1932)
Pascal, Constance and J. Royer, 'La joie qui guérit', *L'Hygiène mentale,* XXXe année, 8, (September–October 1935), 157–65
Paulhan, Frédéric, *La Fonction de la mémoire et le souvenir affectif* (Paris: Alcan, 1904)
Pelletier, Madeleine, *Les Femmes peuvent-elles avoir du génie?* (Paris: n.d.)
— 'Le féminisme et ses militantes', *Documents du progrès* (July 1909), 19–26
Perrot, Michelle, 'Madeleine Pelletier ou le refus de devenir femme', in Christine Bard (ed.), *Madeleine Pelletier: logique et infortunes d'un combat pour l'égalité* (Paris: Côté Femmes, 1992), 185–92
Phillips, Roderick, *Putting Asunder: A History of Divorce in Western Society* (Cambridge: Cambridge University Press, 1988)
Piéron, Henri, 'Une adaptation biologique de Freudisme aux psychonévroses de guerre: l'instinct et l'inconscient de Rivers', *Journal de psychologie normale et pathologique* (1921), 65–76

Poirier, Jacques and R. Natron, 'L'accession des femmes à la carrière médicale (à la fin du XIXe siècle)', *Médecine et philosophie* (Créteil: Cahiers de l'Institut de recherche universitaire, 1981), 82–97

Porter, Roy, *Madness: A Brief History* (Oxford: Oxford University Press, 2002)

Postel, Jacques and Claude Quétel, *Nouvelle histoire de la psychiatrie* (Paris: Dunod, 1983)

Quétel, Claude, *History of Syphilis* [*Le Mal de Naples: histoire de la syphilis*] (1986), trans. by Judith Braddock and Brian Pike (London: Polity Press, 1993)

Recueil Sirey, *Recueil général des lois et des arrêts, ordonnances de 29 novembre 1820, 20 janvier* (Paris: Recueil Dalloz Sirey, 1832)

Rees, Jeanne Pascal, 'À propos de Constance Pascal, première femme aliéniste en France', *L'Information psychiatrique* 2 (February 2001), 173–84

— 'Maladie et mort de Constance Pascal, June–December, 1937' (2003), MS, PRFP

— 'Recollections of Jeanne Streicher', MS, PRFP

Renaut, M.-H., 'Le droit et l'enfant adultérin de l'époque romaine à aujourd'hui, *Revue historique* (1997), 369–408

Ribot, Théodule, *Les Maladies de la mémoire*, (Paris: Germer Beullière, 1881)

— *Les Maladies de la personnalité* (Paris: Germer Beullière, 1885)

— *La Psychologie des sentiments* (Paris: Alcan, 1896)

— *Essai sur les passions* (Paris: Alcan, 1907)

— *Problèmes de psychologie affective* (Paris: Alcan, 1910)

Ricou, Georges, 'Dans les cloîtres de la folie: la Doctoresse Pascal', *Le Petit Journal* (1 January 1933), PRFP

Ripa, Yannick, *Women and Madness: the Incarceration of Women in Nineteenth-century France* (Cambridge: Polity Press, 1986)

Roberts, Mary Louise, *Civilization without Sexes: Reconstructing Gender in Post-War France, 1917–1927* (Chicago and London: University of Chicago Press, 1994)

— *Disruptive Acts: The New Woman in Fin-de-Siècle France* (Chicago and London: University of Chicago Press, 2002)

Rochet, André, 'La situation des asiles de la Seine pendant la guerre, et les transferts des aliénés parisiens en province', *Le Progrès médicale* (25 Octobre 1919), 428–29

Rogues de Fursac et Constance Pascal, 'Adipose douloureuse chez un dément précoce', *L'Encéphale* 1 (1908), 131–138

Rollet-Echalier, Catherine, *La Politique à l'égard de la petite enfance sous la Troisième République* (Paris: Presses Universitaires Françaises, 1990)

Roubaud, Louis, 'Démons et déments', *Détective* (1932), PRFP

Roudinesco, Elisabeth, *La Bataille de cent ans: histoire de la psychanalyse en France* (Paris: Ramsay, vol. 1: Seuil, vol. 2, 1982–86)

Sabbatini, Renato M. E., 'The history of shock therapy in psychiatry', *Brain and Mind Magazine* (December 1997, March 1998)

Samra, Martine Bonvoisin and M. Maignien, *La Presse féminine* (Paris: Presses Universitaires de France, 1986)

Schellenberg, Walter, *The Schellenberg Memoirs*, original German manuscript trans. and ed. Louis Hagen (London: André Deutsch, 1956)

Schultze, Caroline, *La Femme-médecin au XIXe siècle* (Paris: Ollier-Henry, 1888)

Scull, Andrew, *Museums of Madness: the Social Organization of Insanity in nineteenth-century England* (London: Allen Lane, 1979)

Serman, William, *Les Officiers français dans la nation 1814–1914* (Paris: Aubier Montaigne, 1982)

Segal, Naomi, 'Witnessing through the skin: the hysteric's body as text', *Journal of Romance Studies* 9 (3) (2009), 73–85

Seton-Watson, Robert W., *A History of the Romanians from Roman Times to the Completion of Unity* (Cambridge: Cambridge University Press, 1934)

Shorter, Edward P., *Historical Dictionary of Psychiatry* (Oxford: Oxford University Press, 2005)

Shorter, Edward P. and David Healy, *Shock Therapy: A History of Electroconvulsive Treatment in Mental Illness* (Rutgers: Rutgers University Press, 2007)

Skinner, Quentin, *The Return of Grand Theory in the Human Sciences* (Cambridge: Cambridge University Press, 1985)

Sowerwine, Charles, 'Madeleine Pelletier (1874–1939), femme, médecin, militante', *Histoire de la psychiatrie, L'Information psychiatrique* 9 (November 1988), 1183–93

Sowerwine, Charles and C. Maignien, *Madeleine Pelletier, une féministe dans l'arène politique* (Paris: Éditions Ouvrières, 1992)

Stricker, Rémy, *Robert Schumann: le musicien et la folie* (Paris: Gallimard, 1984)

Sullerot, Evelyne, *La Presse féminine* (Paris: Armand Colin, 1966)

Tadié, Jean Yves, *Marcel Proust, Biographie* (Paris: Gallimard, 1996).

Taylor, Robert, *Robert Schumann: His Life and Work* (London: Granada, 1982)

Temperley, Harold W. V., ed., *A History of the Peace Conference of Paris* (6 volumes), (London: Hodder and Stoughton, 1920–24)
Téry, Andrée, 'Comment les sœurs traitent les fous', *La Fronde* (20 January 1902)
— 'Toujours l'hominisme', *La Fronde* (2 December 1902)
— 'Les femmes et l'internat', *La Fronde* (4 December 1902)
Thomas, Gregory M., 'Open psychiatric services in interwar France', *History of Psychiatry* 15 (2) (2004), 131–53
Tillet, Claude, 'Le Centre Hospitalier Spécialisé de Clermont de l'Oise de 1790 à nos jours', *Mémoires de la Société Archéologique et Historique de Clermont en Beauvais* XXXV (1983)
Tomkiewicz, Stanislas, *Les Handicapés de la prime enfance: aspects économiques, sociaux et médicaux* (Paris: Presses Universitaires de France, 1985)
Toulouse, Édouard, 'La femme et les fonctions publiques' (n.d.) Dossier Madeleine Pelletier, BMD
Treptow, Kurt W. (ed.) *The History of Romania* (Iasi: Centre for Romanian Studies, 1997)
Turkle, Sherry, *Psychoanalytic Politics: Freud's French Revolution* (London: Deutsch, 1979)
Vié, Jacques, 'Mademoiselle C. Pascal (1877–1937)', *La Presse médicale* (January 1938), 150
— 'Mademoiselle C. Pascal, Médecin en chef des Hôpitaux Psychiatriques de la Seine, 1877–1937', MS, PRFP
— 'Nécrologie Mlle C. Pascal (1877–1937)', *Annales médico-psychologiques*, 2 (1937), 788 et 868
Weil, Patrick, *La France et ses étrangers* (Paris: Gallimard, 1991)
Weiss, John H, 'Origins of the French welfare state: poor relief in the Third Republic, 1871–1914', *French Historical Studies* XIII (1) (1983), 47–77
Witz, Anne, *Professions and Patriarchy* (London: Routledge, 1992)
Young, Robert, *Mind, Brain and Adaptation in the Nineteenth Century* (Oxford: Oxford University Press, 1970)
Zeldin, Theodore, *France 1848–1945: vol. 2* (Oxford: Oxford University Press, 1970)
Zola, Emile, *L'Assommoir* (1877), trans. Leonard Hancock (Harmondsworth: Penguin, 1970)

Index

www.ingramcontent.com/pod-product-compliance
Lightning Source LLC
LaVergne TN
LVHW012052300826
846742LV00017B/59